D1799772

MASSAGE

STEWART MITCHELL, an experienced clinician and trainer, is director of The School of Complementary Therapies in Exeter, in the UK. He studied Nature Cure methods in Edinburgh, India and the USA, is a certified Health Educator and holds a degree in Complementary Health Studies from the University of Exeter, where he researched the effects of essential oils. He is the author of *The Complete Illustrated Guide to Massage* and *Health Essentials: Naturopathy*, also published by Element.

New Perspectives

THE SERIES

New Perspectives provide attractive and accessible introductions to a comprehensive range of mind, body and spirit topics. Beautifully designed and illustrated, these practical books are written by experts in each subject.

Titles in the series include:

ALEXANDER TECHNIQUE
by Richard Brennan

AROMATHERAPY
by Christine Wildwood

DREAMS
by David Fontana

FENG SHUI
by Man-Ho Kwok with Joanne O'Brien

FLOWER REMEDIES
by Christine Wildwood

HOMEOPATHY
by Peter Adams

MASSAGE
by Stewart Mitchell

MEDITATION
by David Fontana

NLP
by Carol Harris

NUMEROLOGY
by Rodford Barrat

REFLEXOLOGY
by Inge Dougans

TAROT
by A T Mann

New Perspectives

MASSAGE

An Introductory Guide to the Healing Power of Touch

STEWART MITCHELL

ELEMENT

Shaftesbury, Dorset • Boston, Massachusetts
Melbourne, Victoria

© Element Books Limited 1999
Text © Stewart Mitchell 1992, 1999

First published as *Health Essentials: Massage*
in 1992 by Element books Limited

This revised edition first published in Great Britain
in 1999 by Element Books Limited
Shaftesbury, Dorset SP7 8BP

Published in the USA in 1999 by
Element Books, Inc.
160 North Washington Street,
Boston, MA 02114

Published in Australia in 1999 by
Element Books and distributed by
Penguin Australia Limited
487 Maroondah Highway,
Ringwood, Victoria 3134

Designed for Element Books Limited by
Design Revolution, Queens Park Villa,
30 West Drive, Brighton, East Sussex BN2 2GE

ELEMENT BOOKS LIMITED
Editorial Director: Sarah Sutton
Editorial manger: Jane Pizzy
Commissioning Editor: Grace Cheetham
Production Director: Roger Lane

DESIGN REVOLUTION
Editorial Director: Ian Whitelaw
Art Director: Lindsey Johns
Editor: Julie Whitaker
Designer: Vanessa Good

Printed and bound in Great Britain by
Bemrose Security Printing, Derby

British Library Cataloguing in Publication
data available

Library of Congress Cataloging in Publication
data available

ISBN 1-86204-626-3

CONTENTS

FOREWORD

I have known Stewart Mitchell for ten years as a gifted practitioner and have personal experience of his great skill in massage.

It is good that he also teaches massage, because it is a largely neglected but very effective therapeutic tool. The German word for medical treatment is behandlung, which translated literally means "handling". This instructive wisdom of language hints at the healing properties of the hands and links up with the "laying on of hands" in spiritual forms of healing. Stewart has made a careful study of the manifold aspects and benefits of massage – and I am particularly pleased that massage as self-aid and "mutual help" among family and friends has been investigated as separate from professional massage. In this kind of giving the giver is twice blessed, for we hear so many times that those who massage their friends begin to feel much better themselves.

The chapters are carefully designed so that readers can find at a glance the aspects which are of particular importance to them. I trust that this book will fulfil a real need, and I wish it well!

It is also good to know that Stewart has many years ahead of both teaching and protecting this valuable form of therapy in his friendly and truly nourishing centre in Exeter.

DR GORDON LATTO MB CHB

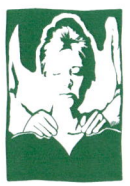

ORIGINS OF MASSAGE

Massage is perhaps one of the most popular forms of health activity today. It is effectively used in relaxation groups and workshops, in leisure centres and as a form of natural therapy for injury. Practised since ancient times, it offers the experience of touch, movement and energy to promote both physical and emotional well-being.

7

THE HISTORY OF MASSAGE

From studies of the classics, it would appear that the ancient Chinese, Greeks and Romans all practised a form of massage. Indeed, a word for massage exists in most cultures. In some societies massage has been used socially as an act of hospitality, such as in Hawaii where passive movements called *lomi-lomi* are bestowed on honoured guests. Aesthetically, the ancient Greeks associated physical culture with the unfolding of mental and spiritual faculties and set up massage schools in their centres of health, which were known as gymnasiums. In the Far East, performing musicians and actors have always learned massage practices to aid their artistic development, while exponents of kathakali, an early dance form originating in South India, are treated with deep massage from the feet of their teachers.

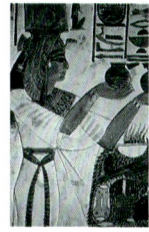

ABOVE ANCIENT EGYPTIAN ART SHOWS THAT THEY PRACTISED MASSAGE WITH OILS.

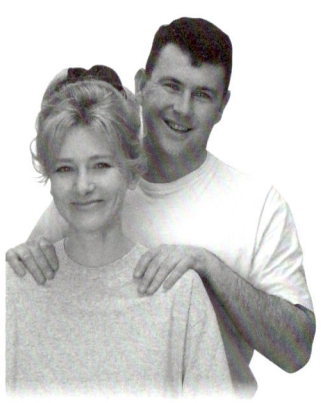

LEFT TODAY MASSAGE IS VERY POPULAR AS PEOPLE LOOK FOR NEW WAYS TO RELIEVE STRESS.

EARLY THERAPEUTIC MASSAGE

Working with only limited concepts of how the body works, early physicians were able to use massage effectively in treating fatigue, illness and injury. Indeed Hippocrates described anatripsis, which means literally 'rubbing up', as having a better effect than rubbing down in the limbs, although a proper understanding of the blood's circulation was at that time incomplete.

It is thought that the development of massage was interrupted with the disintegration of the Greek and Roman civilizations, although an unbroken tradition continued in the East. Not until the 16th century and the emergence of relatively sophisticated surgical techniques in France do we hear of massage re-emerging in Europe in connection with healing.

In the late 19th century the demand for therapeutic massage brought about the formation of societies of therapists, with the objects of organizing training, promoting the science of massage and 'safeguarding the interests of the public and the profession'. Among the qualities needed by a suitable practitioner in 1894 by the Incorporated Society of Massage were 'health', 'intelligence and aptitude', as well as 'a high moral tone'.

MASSAGE TODAY

The popularity of massage in contemporary times is in part a response to the highly stressful conditions of modern life. The reaction against unacceptably dehumanizing elements in healthcare in particular has encouraged the revival of therapies that had been discarded in the scientific age.

However, enthusiasm for massage still meets with resistance today. Massage has been abused socially and there can sometimes be confusion about its place in healing; there remains, too, ignorance and misunderstanding of the body.

THE IMPORTANCE OF TOUCH

Massage is a very sensitive and sensitizing form of human contact, whose medium is touch, a sense to which human beings are especially responsive. Among the animals we have one of the longest infancies, during which time we are dependent on safe handling for protection and guidance in the world around us.

The experience of massage could be said to begin from birth, as the muscles of the uterus deliver the baby along the birth canal by rhythmic contraction. After we are born, holding, rocking, washing and caressing by the parent prepares our body for its independence.

9

As we become more self-controlled, the body's own massage movements become stronger; the movements of our arms and legs against the earth, for example, get us around but are also necessary to help our blood circulate effectively; and the

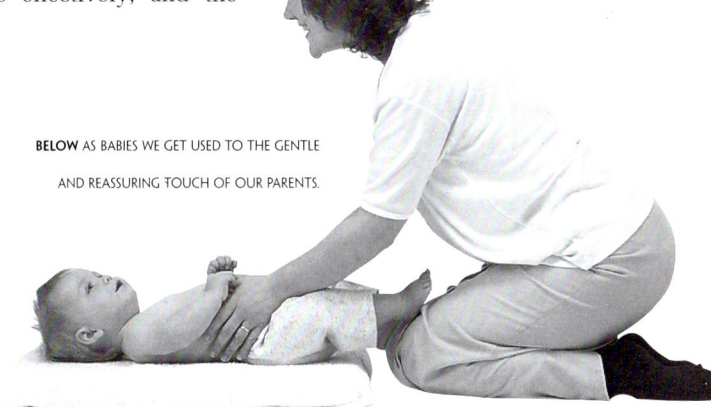

BELOW AS BABIES WE GET USED TO THE GENTLE AND REASSURING TOUCH OF OUR PARENTS.

gradual co-ordination of our hands enables us to squeeze and scratch and soothe ourselves from discomfort.

Emotionally, too, as the early Greeks suspected, the quality of our physical contact with the world is very stimulating. While in the womb, we are well protected and our senses are assumed to be dormant; after birth, while we are acquiring knowledge about sounds, focusing our gaze and recognizing smells, we are particularly dependent on the reassurance of touch. Modern research has indicated that given the choice between food and comforting touch with no food, the infant is more likely to choose touch.

Thus our connection with the origins of massage can be appreciated as much more immediately personal than a historical perspective suggests; the movements of external, given massage are powerful reminders of the security of touch for the adult.

PROFESSIONAL COURSES

It should come as no surprise, therefore, that those who take up massage find that they have a natural aptitude for it. Massaging is an activity in which coaching rather than teaching is called for. You may be cautious about attending courses introducing the principles of massage, which can range from the basic to the esoteric, but their usefulness is to bring you into contact with others and extend your experience. A good course is one in which you feel safe.

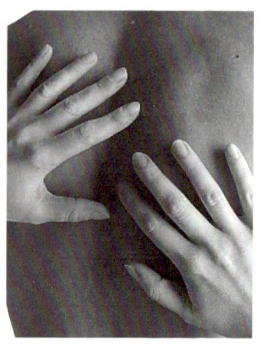

ABOVE A 'HANDS ON' APPROACH TO MASSAGE IS THE BEST WAY TO LEARN ITS TECHNIQUES.

While supporting you to become an original practitioner of massage, this book does not discourage formal massage between professional and client; in fact I recommend that you take advantage of, and support, professional practices that may be available to you. I'm sure you will find that contact with a therapist becomes increasingly helpful as your own massage skills evolve.

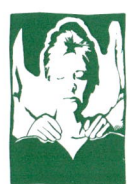

MASSAGE FOR PLEASURE, EXERCISE AND HEALTH

CHAPTER TWO

Being healthy helps us to be happy, energetic and purposeful. It is generally accepted that we can become healthier by following athletic and creative pursuits, or by modifying those aspects of our behaviour that are thought to be harmful. A contrasting approach is that health is not a state that can be achieved but an attitude towards life, not struggling for what is already ours. So what is 'health'?

APPROACHES TO HEALTH

'Are health and fitness the same?' is a reasonable question, often discussed in leisure centres. The frenetic pursuit of health can be confused with the fear of illness, and guilt from all our unhealthy habits. For some, health may be related to the achievement of personal goals, yet many outstanding athletes

RIGHT KEEPING FIT CAN CERTAINLY HELP IN ONE'S QUEST FOR HEALTH, BUT IT IS NOT ONLY THE BODY BUT THE MIND THAT THE PRACTICE OF MASSAGE ADDRESSES.

and artists have not possessed perfect health; high achievers often speak of the emotional strain of success and the pressures that accompany it. At the other extreme, advice to conform to safe, restrictive practices in the way we eat, drink and proceed in life is not universally convincing – it is rarely disputed that too much dietary fat damages blood vessels, that smoking irritates the lungs or that constant worrying depletes nerves, but avoiding these behaviours does not appear to insure us against ill-health.

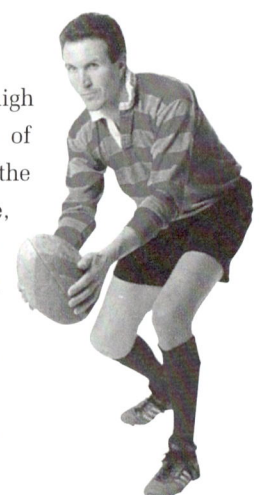

MIND AND BODY

Are there individual qualities of health that enable some people to retain an integrated body and mind, be it in success or failure, in

ABOVE THE HIGH GOALS THAT TOP SPORTS PLAYERS SET THEMSELVES CAN LEAD TO EMOTIONAL STRAIN.

occasional excess or in conserving themselves? Perhaps we can be inspired by those who, towards the end of their lives, say why they feel so satisfied. Not infrequently we hear of their inquisitiveness, their enthusiasm to take risks and become involved in life, without any apparent confidence.

In this book we are going to begin, perhaps tentatively, an appreciation of health by observing, investigating and experimenting with massage. Take a moment to realize that this will be a serious adventure, in that it could bring you some direct, tangible benefits; at the same time, it's likely to be a really pleasurable experience!

MOVEMENT AND THE HEALTHY BODY

Movement is often regarded as a sign of life; it is certainly an indication of health. This is true not only of speed or strength but especially in co-ordination, since a well co-ordinated body usually feels as good as it looks.

Most of our routine physical tasks are unconsciously directed, yet all were patiently learned. Seemingly effortless movements, however, can revert to clumsiness as soon as we become tired or nervous. How often do we miss the last step or trip on the first and experience a real shock! We don't congratulate ourselves on achieving simple tasks and yet we are indignant when we fail; we take the skill of our movement for granted, including the satisfaction that it gives. We only fully appreciate our mobility when we lose it and perhaps for this reason someone who develops a bad back or a stiff neck can be difficult to live with.

INVOLUNTARY MOVEMENT

Some of our most complicated movements take place inside the body, strictly un-conscious and beyond our voluntary control: the circulation of the blood, propulsion of food through the intestines, and erection of body hairs for example. Curiously, these move-ments are accomplished equally effectively by the lazy as they are by the fit. This is because the effort comes from what we are made up of as well as what we do with ourselves. It can explain why some people appear to maintain their health in spite of their habits rather than by trying to be healthy.

13

LEFT MANY PEOPLE TAKE THE ABILITY TO MOVE AND
PERFORM SIMPLE PHYSICAL TASKS FOR GRANTED –
THAT IS UNTIL AN INJURY, SUCH AS A BAD BACK, OCCURS.

GET IN TOUCH WITH YOUR BODY

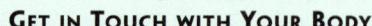

For children, having a body is exciting – it's new! Our early activities are full of surprises; even our mistakes, such as dropping things and falling over, are fun, and we don't feel the pain or embarrassment this can cause us as adults. In adulthood we are tenser and have much more to lose from our errors. We pay the price for this tension with a diminished sense of fun. How relaxed are you with your own sense of movement? As an exercise, try crawling around the room on all fours as you once did as a child, or see how long you can stand on one leg. How do you feel doing this? Uncomfortable? Afraid? Or do you get a sneaking sense of relief from the strain of being grown-up?

ABOVE AND RIGHT AS YOU LEARN ABOUT MASSAGE, YOUR INTIMACY WITH YOUR OWN BODY WILL INCREASE AND YOU MAY REGAIN THE SENSE OF WONDER AND FUN YOU EXPERIENCED AS A CHILD.

14

OUR AMAZING HANDS

Take a good look at your hands and move them gently. In spite of any personal reservations you might have, from the point of view of structure, sensitivity and aesthetics, your hands are unsurpassed. They contain the ability to

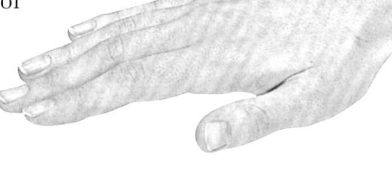

ABOVE YOUR HANDS ARE INCREDIBLY SENSITIVE WITH NUMEROUS NERVE ENDINGS, MAKING THEM IDEAL MASSAGE TOOLS.

perform incredible tasks. Interestingly, you may have noticed that there are few muscles in the hand: wriggle your fingers while watching your forearms, and you will notice your finger bones are operated from a distance by arm muscles, like puppetry. Otherwise the constant movement of muscular hands would make them grow too big for their delicate manipulations.

Are you equally familiar with both hands? How many bones can you count in your fingers? How do you explain that your hand can turn a door handle without your body doing a cartwheel?

HAND-EYE CO-ORDINATION

Together with all their skills of dexterity, hands have great powers of sense, having amongst the most numerous of nerve endings of any part of the skin. The eyes are dependent on the hands to confirm reality. Our early development of hand-eye co-ordination is very important, and later in life if we are plunged into darkness our hands reliably take over. Asked how they would negotiate a darkened room, people might say by sound or echo or by visualizing previous impressions, but quite probably their hands would immediately be reaching out – recognizing, guiding and solving the problem.

This book presents the opportunity to realize just how much our hands can be relied upon therapeutically. Our hands are there as the tools and the means to encourage our bodies to health.

HOW THE BODY MASSAGES ITSELF

Even if the idea of massage might be attractive, enjoyment of a massage is not something that is immediately acceptable to everyone. There are many reasons for this, not least that if you were not handled agreeably as a child, you are unlikely to trust being handled as an adult. Fortunately, the body is designed in such a way as to be constantly massaging itself and this can give us some confidence to begin with.

- The diaphragm muscle between the chest and abdomen alternately compresses and releases the digestive organs with each deep breath.

- Even the slightest movement of the limb muscles squeezes and relieves pressure on the nearby veins to keep peripheral circulation flowing.

- The arms, kept free to swing by the sides as we walk, relax the muscles of the back.

THE BODY'S NATURAL DEFENCE SYSTEM

A minor injury such as a fall or even an argument can lead to a localized painful stiffening of the muscles and joints and is one of the body's natural defence responses. Stiffening has the overall effect of providing time to process a response and generate flexibility. If the experience was a physical confrontation, you can prepare in anticipation of the next time. If, however the experience was emotional, you have the time to rehearse a response mentally.

MASSAGE FOR THE TIRED BODY

1   When you are unwell or tired, many of your natural body movements become depressed. You may notice that if you have to sit still over a long period of time your lower legs seem to 'fill up'. If you've slipped your shoes off, as you might do on a long journey, they will probably feel harder to put back on. This is because the natural massaging movements of the legs have been inhibited by sitting still, and the effect of gravity is slowing down the extreme circulations. Unremedied, this situation may induce a headache or drowsiness. After a few minutes of simple massage movements, of wringing and stroking, the situation can be eased and the whole body will feel more comfortable.

2   Many people will have experienced the stiffening, locally or over a larger area of the body, which comes after a collision or fall or even an unpleasant emotional exchange. Muscles and joints that normally glide effortlessly under the skin become painfully stiff and the person's tense posture will reflect this. Here massage intervention can be valuable by not only easing and loosening our condition but also creating a reassuring atmosphere within the body.

RIGHT IN EVERYDAY SITUATIONS, SIMPLE SELF-MASSAGE STROKES CAN RELIEVE PAINFUL PROBLEMS SUCH AS ANKLES THAT ARE SWOLLEN THROUGH INACTIVITY.

17

INVITATION TO HEALTH

To maintain or recover health it is possible to have treatment or perhaps to study health or read books about it. The exciting and rewarding possibilities of massage are that it offers a combination of these approaches. You receive physical and mental benefits both in giving and receiving massage. In fact 'health' may take on a whole new meaning for you. People new to massage often express delight in their rediscovery of touch and movement – as receivers, in their capacity to respond, and in giving, in the heightened awareness of their own touch and creativity.

The material for this book is drawn directly from treatments and classwork that people have found to be useful and enjoyable. In both treating and teaching, I have found the acquisition of specific techniques secondary to the development of sensitivity; consequently, the theme of this book is how the appreciation and enjoyment of health is already in our hands.

18

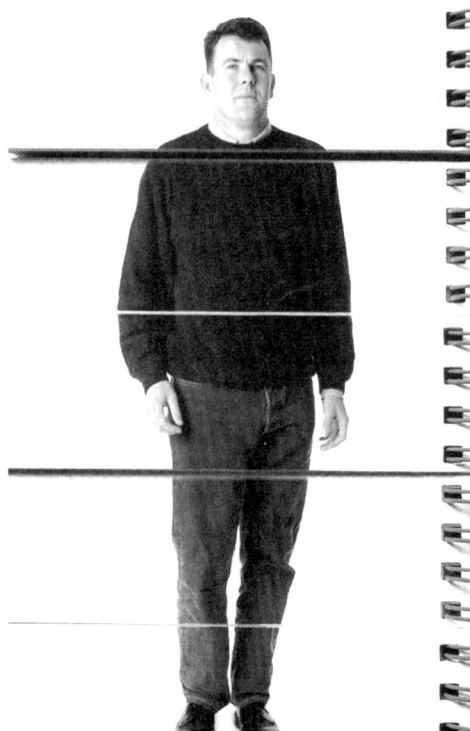

RIGHT THE MANY HEALTH BENEFITS OF MASSAGE CAN BE FELT THROUGHOUT THE WHOLE BODY.

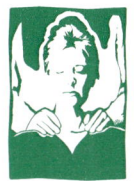

UNDERSTANDING YOUR BODY

Compared with other creatures, the human body may not be as elegant, fast or strong but it is by far the most complex and is a fascinating subject for study. Indeed, learning about the basic structure of your body is essential for anyone who wants to learn how to massage sensitively and especially so if you ever use massage as a form of treatment for injury or illness.

ANATOMY OF MOVEMENT

Our external movements are created by muscles consciously working in conjunction with bones, while internally the muscular system creates heat and stimulates the circulation of blood, digestion and respiratory processes. Even when apparently at rest, the muscles vibrate in anticipation of movement. This enables you to jump into

RIGHT THE WAY OUR MUSCLES WORK IS CRUCIAL TO HOW WE MOVE. RELIEVING TENSION FROM MUSCLES IS ONE OF THE MAJOR BENEFITS OF MASSAGE.

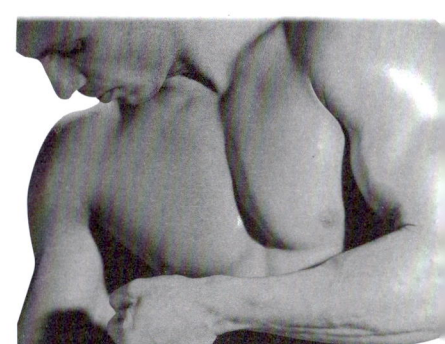

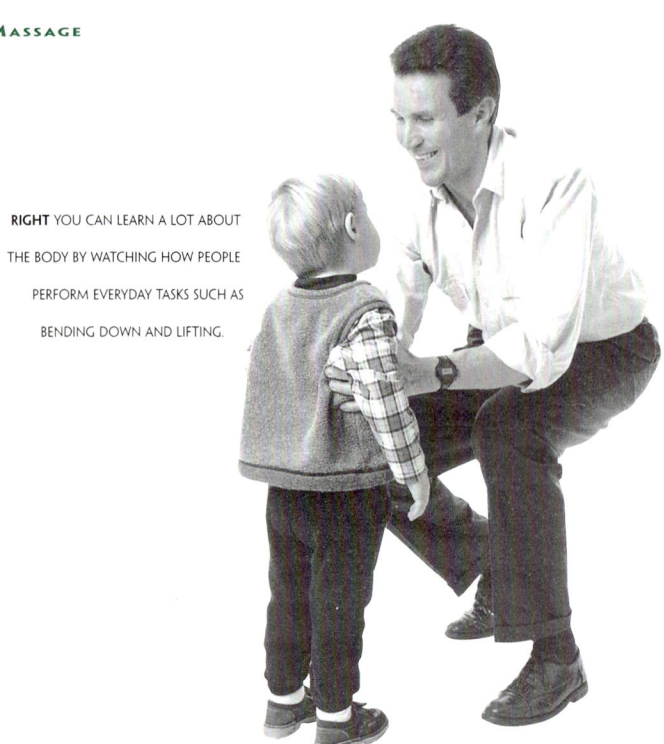

RIGHT YOU CAN LEARN A LOT ABOUT
THE BODY BY WATCHING HOW PEOPLE
PERFORM EVERYDAY TASKS SUCH AS
BENDING DOWN AND LIFTING.

action at extremely short notice, whether, for example, to avert
danger or to eject a morsel of food that has found its way into your
windpipe. You can learn a great deal about the body from observing
everyday movements. Notice the different ways people get in or out
of cars or catch falling objects. Knowledge gained this way is just as
relevant to massage as reading about muscle action.

THE SPINAL COLUMN

The spinal column is the pivotal structure for all movement and,
together with your developed buttock muscles, distinguishes your
posture from that of other creatures. Curiously, we have come to
regard our buttocks as seats, when in fact these muscles are primarily
responsible for our ability to stand upright for long periods. This is in
contrast to a kangaroo, for example, which needs a long flat tail for
upright balance, and even apes are obliged to drop down on to their

knuckles occasionally – we have the freedom to use our upper limbs for more sophisticated purposes. Although strong and flexible, the spine is vulnerable to habitual postures that unbalance its tensions.

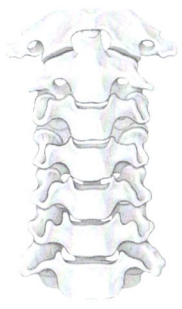

Located close to the centre of the body, all the postural muscles are attached to it, so bad practices such as slumping at your desk or habitually crossing your legs can throw it out of alignment.

THE LOWER BACK

The muscles of your lower back are not easily strained, in spite of the great tensions

ABOVE WHILE ONE END OF THE SPINE IS UNDER STRESS FROM THE LEGS, THE OTHER, THE NECK, HAS TO MAINTAIN THE POSTURE OF THE HEAD.

that can accumulate there, unless you lift yourself (and sometimes even the lightest object) awkwardly.

21

If your back 'goes', it is more likely to be a muscular response than the infamous disc, which does not actually 'slip'. Human evolution is then temporarily reversed and your first reaction is probably to drop forward on to your hands so as to take the weight of the body from the spine; relief usually comes from lying on your back as flat as possible.

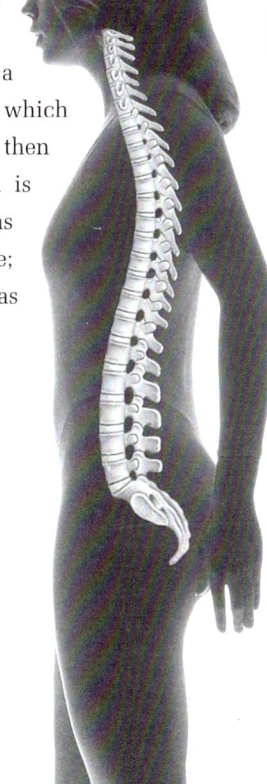

RIGHT THE SPINAL COLUMN HAS 33 RING-LIKE BONES CALLED VERTEBRAE THAT ARE STACKED ONE UPON THE OTHER AND THAT RUN FROM THE NECK TO THE LUMBAR REGION.

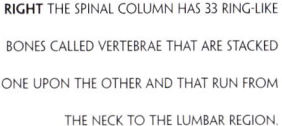

THE BONES

Your bones are known collectively as the skeleton, which means 'dried up'. They are extremely dynamic and versatile structures that are not only concerned with movement but also provide protection for organs such as the brain, as well as being involved in the production of blood cells. Bones are very light yet extremely strong, and like scaffolding poles can withstand great stress. If a simple fracture occurs, the bone's healing is usually so complete that it is unlikely that it will break again at the same point. General massage of the remainder of the body is beneficial while fractures are immobilized for healing, and very supportive when your partner is regaining the use of a healed bone.

RIGHT AN ADULT HAS A TOTAL OF 206 BONES CONNECTED BY JOINTS. OUR BONES ARE QUITE SOFT WHEN WE ARE BORN, BUT HARDEN BY THE AGE OF 20.

THE MUSCLES

Muscles are everywhere in the body, making up the mass of your weight and shape. Some are easy to locate and have individual names such as the well-known biceps, which help to flex the elbow.

The numerous erector muscles of the body hairs are detected only in their effects, as when the hairs stand on end to keep the heat

LEG CROSSING

Many of us cross our legs when seated, usually with a preference for one leg over the other. However, this common posture is very bad for the spine, since it creates a constant twisting and shortening of the deep pelvic muscles. Often when seated in this way for a long period, one leg will go numb – a sensation that indicates the strain the posture is putting on the spine. Then, as the head tries to remain in a balanced position, despite the twisting of the spine, neck tension and pain can occur. Massage can definitely help here.

RIGHT THE TENDENCY TO CROSS ONE'S LEGS TWISTS THE SPINE AND IS BEST AVOIDED.

23

within the skin. Muscles only contract (i.e. shorten) to cause a movement, and rely on the contraction of their opposite neighbouring muscles to relax out.

You can illustrate this for yourself: Straighten your elbow. If both the biceps (at the front of the upper arm) and the triceps (at the rear) contract simultaneously, the elbow locks straight; when the biceps increases its contraction the triceps agrees to relax and the elbow flexes. Beginning again from this position, try the movement in reverse.

Muscles faithfully record our feelings, and their tensions help ease stressful situations. However, when this tension is not relaxed

MUSCLE FUNCTION

Muscles are responsible for a wonderful range of tasks:

- They give us strength
- They help keep the blood warm
- They cushion us
- They reliably guard against collisions with our environment. For example, if we should fall over we would be wise to let the larger muscles take the impact rather than an outstretched hand and risk an arm fracture.

24

sufficiently, the lining of the muscles and surrounding tissues are irritated, creating the classic condition known as fibrositis. Almost everyone has had this experience of tension, and massage is justly famous for alleviating it.

RIGHT OUR MUSCLES ARE RESPONSIBLE FOR THE WAY OUR BODY MOVES. THERE ARE 650 MUSCLES IN THE HUMAN BODY. EVEN WHEN YOU THINK YOU ARE SITTING STILL YOUR MUSCLES CONTINUE TO WORK.

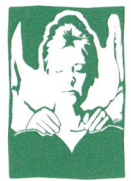

BASIC MASSAGE TECHNIQUES

Although the focal point for massagers tends to be their hands, after a little experience you will begin to appreciate that giving massage involves your whole body: your back muscles hold you poised and accommodate the weight of your partner; your legs transfer your weight and give depth to the treatment; and the upper arms provide the strength for your strokes. It is really important, therefore, that you are physically and mentally prepared for the demands of giving a massage.

AVOIDING PHYSICAL STRAIN

Your aim is to be as relaxed as your partner while giving massage, otherwise your tension may become contagious. To avoid tension and the occupational strains associated with giving massage, it is advisable to consider these aspects of your own anatomy.

RIGHT CORRECT POSITIONING IS IMPORTANT.

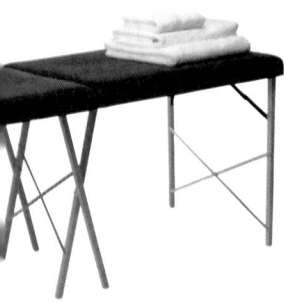

ABOVE THE MASSAGE TABLE SHOULD BE THE CORRECT HEIGHT.

YOUR BACK

To avoid your own back aching in the course of a massage, use the effleurage stroke consistently (*see* p.29), slightly leaning away from your partner. This will stretch out your upper back and, by re-aligning the head with the spine momentarily, lower back pressure is relieved. Occasionally retracting the abdominal muscles and standing as close as you can to the table, with bent knees, will also minimize back strain. Massagers should regularly employ first aid and other self-treating methods (*see* Chapter 8).

YOUR LEGS

Whether you stand or sit to give a massage, the leg muscles are used to give rhythm to your strokes. If your partner is on a couch, stand halfway along, close in, and see if you can comfortably reach their head or feet without moving a step. Bend both knees as you do this and feel how this is also much easier for your back when you are leaning across the table.

If the table is too high and you cannot reach the extremities: make a small running board to massage from, rather than sawing down the legs of the couch, in case you end up with a couch that is too low.

When kneeling, use your thigh muscles to lift and lower your hips when reaching across your partner. A massage stool can be very useful for kneelers who have stiff ankles or cannot take all their weight on their feet.

YOUR ARMS

Pushing and pulling movements are accomplished by muscles that attach the upper arm to the shoulders and chest. To develop your strength, exercises such as push-ups and pull-ups are sometimes recommended. You may have to do these if you find yourself tiring initially, but regular massaging itself creates strength.

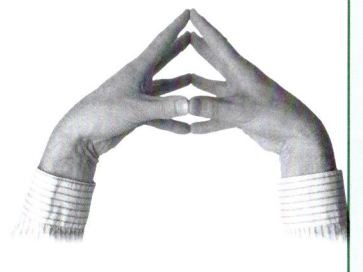

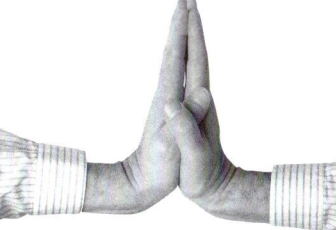

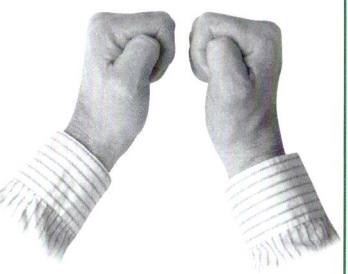

WARM-UP EXERCISES

Before giving a massage, you might like to use these exercises to build strength and suppleness:

1   Widen your elbows and place your fingertips together; press slowly until each finger is stretched flat against its opposite, wrists fully flexed. Lower the hands to increase the stretch.

2   Make fists, then throw out the fingers as wide apart and as straight as possible; hold for 10 seconds and repeat six times.

3   Relax your hands and shake vigorously from the wrists in all directions, keeping your elbows flexed and your arms still. Stop when your hands feel 'rubbery' and your fingers tingle.

27

ABOVE AND RIGHT SUPPLE HANDS HELP YOU TO 'FEEL' YOUR WAY AROUND YOUR PARTNER'S BODY DURING MASSAGE.

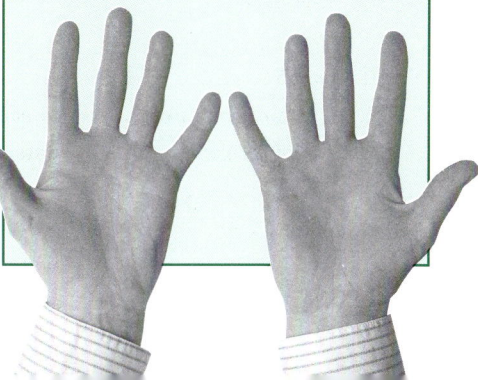

BASIC MASSAGE STROKES

The many different strokes of massage and their unique physical and psychological benefits were rationalized by a Swede, Professor Henry Ling, in the 19th century. His 'Swedish System' was incorporated into medicine but its reputation has suffered both in the popular image of the massage 'parlour' and in its declining use in physiotherapy, which has become more mechanized.

Ling's classical strokes define massage as a combination of three movements, effleurage, petrissage and kneading, and percussion.

EFFLEURAGE

This is the preparatory and background stroke. It is non-invasive since it puts no pressure into the body and does not attempt to move it; this is very important at the beginning and end of a massage. Although superficial in comparison with other strokes, effleurage is profound in its effects due to the skin's nervous connections with

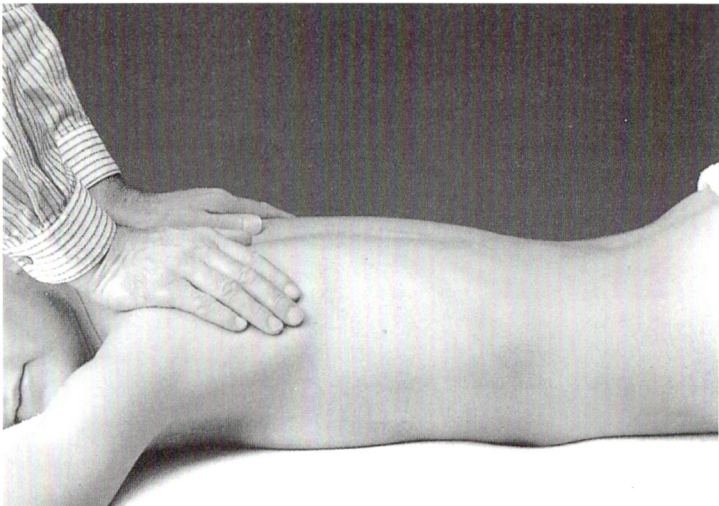

ABOVE PLACE YOUR HANDS LIGHTLY ON YOUR PARTNER'S BACK AND GLIDE THEM DOWN EITHER SIDE OF THE SPINE. AS YOU PERFORM EFFLEURAGE KEEP YOUR ELBOWS STRAIGHT AND MAINTAIN AN EVEN PRESSURE.

deeper parts of the body. For effleurage, lay the whole surface of the palm of your hand on your partner's body and stroke smoothly, following the contours of the body.

- Effleurage is appreciated by slender or anxious partners.
- Effleurage helps you to attune to your partner.

PETRISSAGE

For petrissage, take hold of an edge of the body (for example, the inside thigh) with your fingertips. Move along making squeezing strokes using the balls of your thumbs. This type of pressure is suitable on sinewy muscles found in the limbs and upper back. Petrissage adjusts their tension rather than forcing it out, which they would resist.

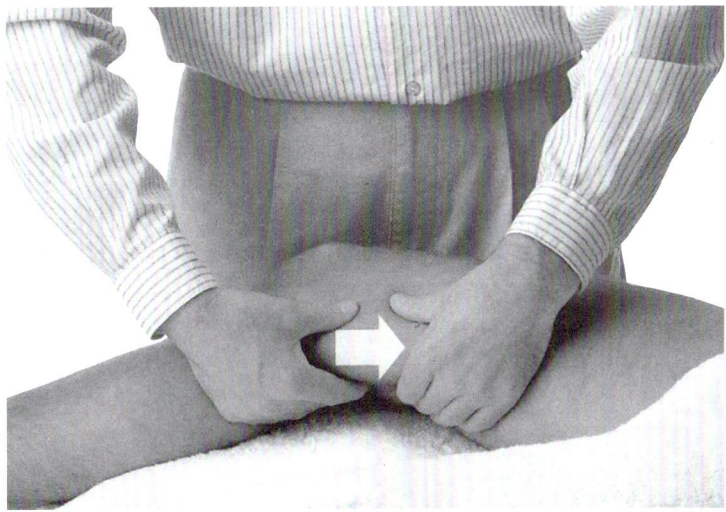

ABOVE THE TECHNIQUE OF PETRISSAGE WORKS WELL ON THE SINEWY MUSCLES OF THE LEG.

- Petrissage allows detailed work on the body.
- Petrissage is recommended on children and older adults.
- Petrissage develops sensitivity in the fingers.

KNEADING

Most people associate massage with the deep stroke, kneading, where curved muscles, such as those on the front of the thigh are squeezed with the whole hand and thumb. This stroke is used to break down deep tensions and condition muscles to have even tension. Encouraging the muscles to be more sponge-like helps local circulation and assists the heart. Depending on the shape of a large muscle, kneading can also be done with the heel of the hand or foot, knuckles or elbow. It is worth noting that the experience can be very emotional because deep tensions are being released.

- Kneading is best suited for partners who are muscular and use their muscles vigorously.
- Kneading requires strength in the arms and thumb muscles, which will develop with practice.
- Kneading can be overdone and both massager and partner will feel tired. When this happens, interrupt with effleurage.

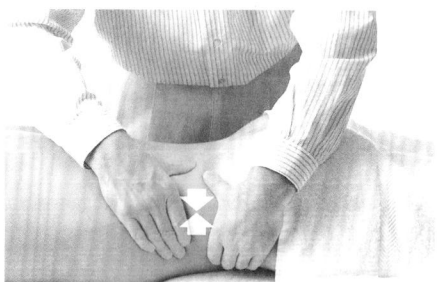

RIGHT FOR THE WAIST, GATHER HANDFULS OF FLESH, AND PASS THEM BETWEEN YOUR HANDS AND THUMBS.

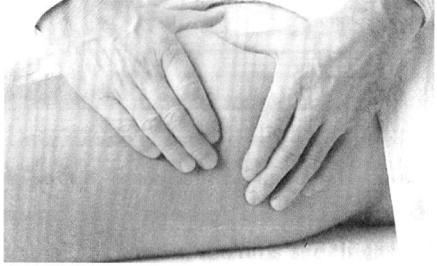

RIGHT TO MASSAGE THE BUTTOCKS, APPLY DEEP PRESSING STROKES USING THE WHOLE OF YOUR HAND.

PERCUSSION

So that those receiving a massage treatment can pick themselves up, feeling relaxed but also ready to face life again, a massage is completed by skilful striking of the body. Ling calls this stroke percussion. It uses wrist movement to stimulate the body with different parts of the hand. Percussion is designed to reintegrate the muscles, lessening the contrast from deep relaxation back into everyday movement. There are three types of percussion stroke: hacking, cupping and tapotement.

HACKING

Hacking is a general percussion performed lightly with the fingers. It causes muscles to 'wake up' without disturbing your partner's sense of relaxation. For hacking, place your palms in a parallel position. Slightly stretch your fingers and chop from the wrist so that the lower three fingers make contact with the body, while vibrating against each other. Hack slowly, then build up speed and depth.

CUPPING

Cupping is used on the lower back and can be helpful over the rib case. It encourages deep circulation in the large muscles and prepares them for action. For cupping, make your hands into a 'cup' that would be watertight; turn upside down and beat the body by alternately flexing the wrists. Begin slowly, maintaining the cup as you increase in speed and depth. You will hear a hollow sound as the air is beaten from the surface of the skin; finger marks on the skin reveal that the cup is too shallow and your partner will be feeling the percussion uncomfortably.

TAPOTEMENT

Tapotement is the lightest percussion, mostly applied around the face and head and sensitive areas. For tapotement, drum your fingertips across the face avoiding contact with the eyes. On larger areas the fingers are kept together and tapped against the skin.

COMMUNICATION DURING MASSAGE

While it is good to have explanations for your work, verbal conversation can often interrupt the feedback from touch. In silence, new sensations arising into consciousness can intercept tensions and allow the benefits of the treatment to last longer. You are certainly not obliged to give a running commentary on your massage and you may occasionally feel that you want to discourage too much questioning from a nervous partner. Changes in tension can bring up feelings of insecurity, however, and although with practice you should be able to anticipate this, be ready to respond verbally if your partner needs reassurance.

32

BELOW DURING MASSAGE,
OUR HANDS HOLD A
CONVERSATION WITH
OUR PARTNER'S
MUSCLES.

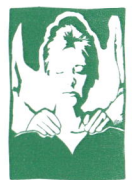

PRACTICAL MASSAGE

CHAPTER FIVE

Most adults approach their first massage with a variety of preconceptions. Regardless of your approach, your partner may expect massage to be an athletic or hedonistic experience, threatening or relaxing, daringly sexual or completely clinical. The actual massage will soon clarify these thoughts. It is crucially important that both of the people involved are equally comfortable with whatever environment you have chosen or created for the experience.

33

SETTING UP

Massages are given in whichever situation seems appropriate. Most professionals have a quiet room and a treatment couch but you might like to use a kitchen table or chair, and some massagers find the floor perfectly suitable.

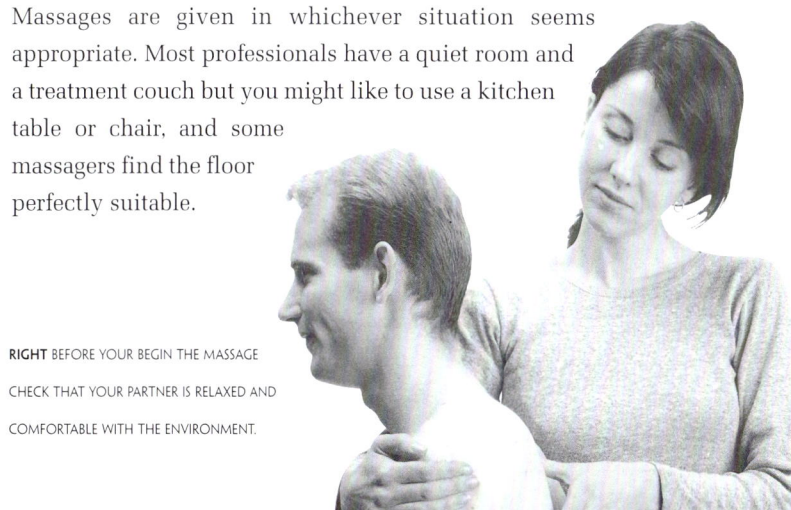

RIGHT BEFORE YOUR BEGIN THE MASSAGE CHECK THAT YOUR PARTNER IS RELAXED AND COMFORTABLE WITH THE ENVIRONMENT.

An issue for your partner will be how he or she is used to being handled, both at present and when he or she was very young. This psychological aspect means that partners are particularly vulnerable to the first and last touch of massage; so make sure that the beginning and ending of your treatments are slow and gentle, careful and reassuring.

EQUIPMENT

You will need several clean towels. Fold one and use it as a head rest and the others to cover the areas of your partner's body that you are not massaging at any one time. For example, if you are working on the limbs, cover the torso with a towel, and then when massaging the torso, move it down to cover the limbs. This will help to keep your partner warm and relaxed during the treatment.

Decide whether you want to use any talc or oil for the massage. Talc can be useful at the beginning of massage, while oil is helpful in detailed work. Anxiety at the early stage of treatment can cause both people to sweat, which makes effleurage difficult, and massage strokes on very dry skin can create uncomfortable friction. Thus you may like to use talc for convenience early in the treatment or for the first massage. Oil massage can be recommended for children and older adults because it deflects too much direct pressure away from the body. Massage to loosen a stiff or painful joint can also be a suitable occasion for utilizing the gliding influence of oil. Add oil a little at a time on to your hand first, rather than direct to the body. However, remember that when you begin to practise massage, the direct contact between your hand and your partner's skin is necessary in recognizing tension and the condition of muscles and an oily or powdery substance may get in the way of your experience of the body.

WHEN NOT TO MASSAGE

You should always make some enquiries about your partner's general health before giving massage. When massage is given for the purpose of relaxation and support, it is very unlikely that someone's medical condition will disqualify him or her from receiving it. If any of the conditions below apply to your partner, keep the strokes well within their comfort.

Has your partner recently:
* Taken regular medication?
* Undergone surgery?
* Had an accident or injury?
* Undergone osteopathic or chiropractic treatment?
* Is your partner pregnant or menstruating?

Although there are serious states of health in which massage is contra-indicated, it is very likely that massage is being denied to more people whose condition would benefit from treatment than could ever be harmed by it. When you are unsure about someone's suitability for treatment, consult an experienced practitioner.

ESSENTIAL OILS

Essential oils, used for aromatherapy, are highly concentrated and very powerful and in some cases are not beneficial during massage. Don't use them on a pregnant woman or during the early stages of breast feeding. A simple rule to follow is not to use oil on someone who doesn't like its aroma – it probably won't do them any good at all. If you or your partner are attracted to aromatherapy, use the oils sparingly and check any possible contra-indications before beginning the treatment.

HAND MASSAGE

A body massage is not necessarily given in any special order but you might like to follow the sequence in this chapter for practice. For someone new to the treatment, hand massage can be a good way to begin as it provides a familiar point of contact and you can look at and talk to each other in the usual way.

The hand is a natural introduction to the rest of the body with its many muscles, joints and varying thickness of skin.

Apart from local soothing benefits, massaging the hands helps to reduce any pressure in the neck and head by nervous and circulatory effects.

MASSAGE TECHNIQUE

1   Have your partner lie down with his or her right arm flexed and resting on the elbow, with a small pillow underneath.

2   Effleurage the hand between your hands, softly squeezing down from the fingertips to the wrist, like a glove being pulled on. Move back to the fingertips with a lighter pressure and repeat the movement 12–20 times.

36

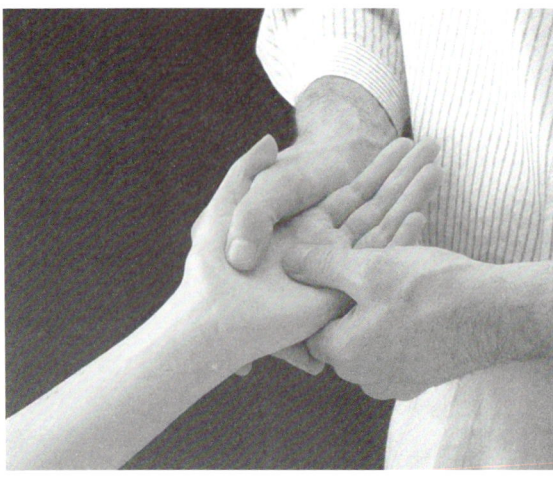

LEFT STEP 4: MAKE SURE YOU GIVE SPECIAL ATTENTION TO YOUR PARTNER'S THUMB.

3 Petrissage by turning the palm downwards, placing your fingertips and thumbs on to the back of the hand, and squeeze all over. Stroke the back of the hand with your thumbs 12 times.

4 Turn the hand upwards and squeeze the palm and base of the thumb.

5 Effleurage as at 2., firmly upwards.

6 Support the hand and percuss it lightly all over with your stiffened fingers.

7 Effleurage lightly.

Place your partner's hand on his or her abdomen, then begin the sequence over again on the other hand.

Congratulations if this is your first massage! Ask your partner for comments and criticisms and tell him or her anything interesting you noticed about the hands, and ask your partner if one hand feels different to the other. Later you may prefer to let your treatments speak for themselves.

37

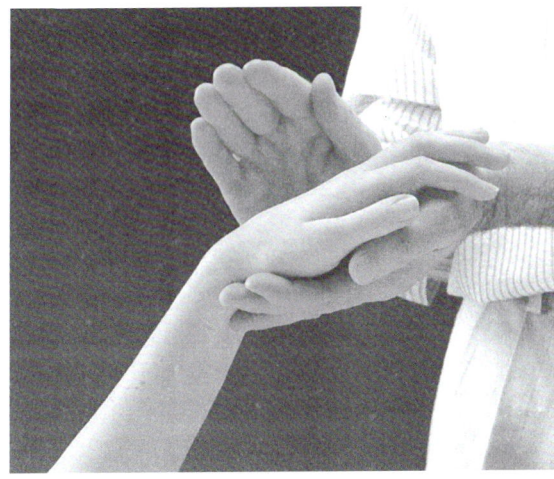

LEFT STEP 6: KEEP YOUR HAND STRAIGHT AND GIVE YOUR PARTNER'S HAND LIGHT BUT SHARP TAPPING MOVEMENTS.

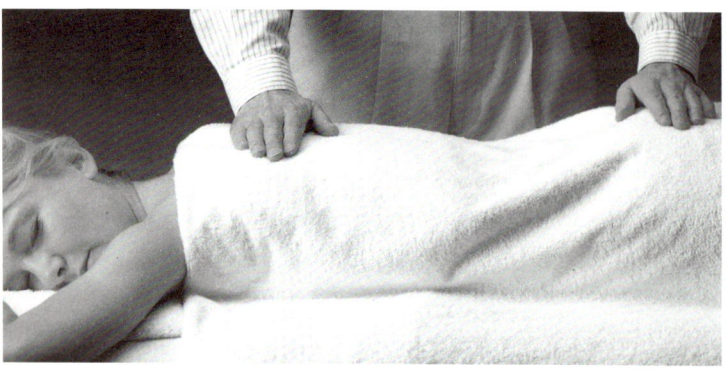

ABOVE COVER YOUR PARTNER WITH TOWELS TO HELP KEEP THE BODY AS WARM AND RELAXED AS POSSIBLE THROUGHOUT THE EXERCISE.

'BREATHING BODY' SEQUENCE

38

A general massage beginning with the back of the trunk is very effective in quickly relaxing the postural muscles. Some partners find it easier to settle into a treatment by not facing the massager.

As an introduction to the back you might like to use this 'Breathing Body' sequence. It creates a calm atmosphere and gives you an opportunity to observe something very subtle about the skeleton.

1   Have your partner lie face down. Place a pillow under the abdomen and feet. The arms can be placed around the head or by the sides of the torso.
2   Place one hand lightly on the middle of the back and the other over the pelvis. Invite your partner to relax and breathe deeply. You will notice the rise and fall of the chest with breathing – can you feel a corresponding, though softer, movement at the pelvis?
3   Remove your hand from the back and place it lightly on the back of the skull. After a few moments the pelvic movement will become more obvious.
4.   Now concentrate on the skull to detect a fainter movement.

Orthodox anatomy teaches that hardly any movement occurs in a stationary pelvis and none at all in the skull; with practice you will become aware that all these areas do actually move in harmony with the breathing.

When you have completed the 'Breathing Body" sequence, you and your partner will feel composed and relaxed, and ready to continue the treatment.

BACK MASSAGE

The complete back massage usually takes 15–20 minutes, certainly not much longer if a whole body treatment is being given. Make use of the respite of effleurage whenever you feel tired.

MASSAGE TECHNIQUE

1 Take up position at your partner's head, facing down the length of the body.

2 Effleurage by gliding softly down the centre of the back with both hands and return via the edges of the body, up to the arms. Repeat 10 times, increasing in depth.

3 Knead using the heels of the hands and the palms to press diagonally across the whole back, up and down, for 30 seconds. Repeat effleurage five times.

4 Move to the side of your partner. Lean over and effleurage the opposite buttock. Knead for 30 seconds. Effleurage deeply in a circular motion. Perform percussion (cupping) on the buttock for approximately 10 seconds. Effleurage lightly.

39

ABOVE STEP 2: AS YOU REPEAT THE EFFLEURAGE SEQUENCE, INCREASE THE DEPTH OF THE STROKES.

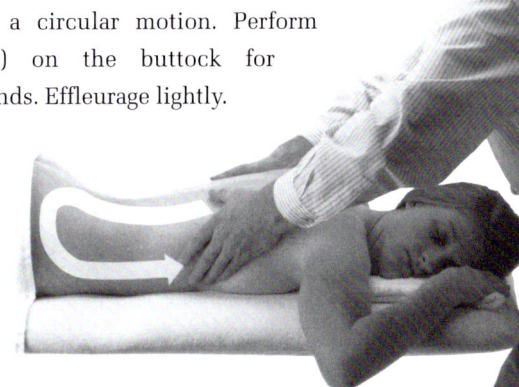

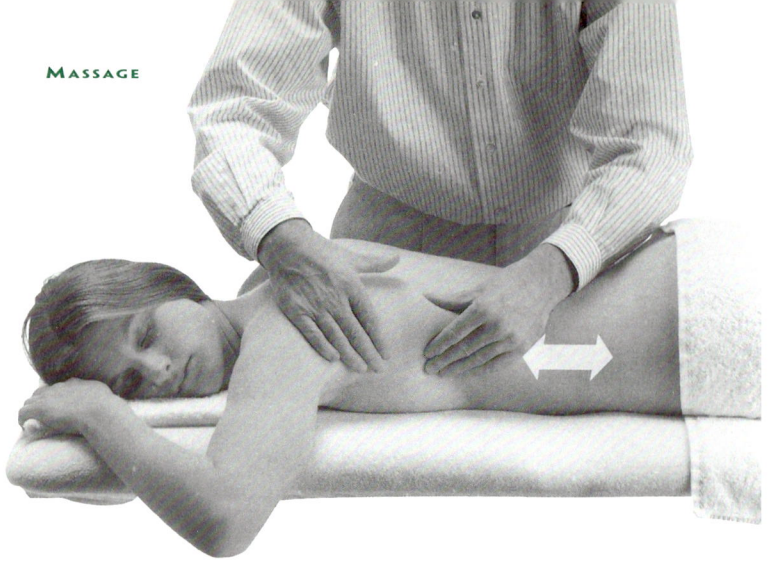

ABOVE STEP 5: IF THIS STROKE TICKLES YOUR PARTNER, DRAW THE ARM CLOSER TO THE SIDE AND BEGIN AGAIN.

5   Effleurage the edge of the chest. Petrissage from the armpit to the waist and back again for 30 seconds. Effleurage deeply towards the armpit. Perform percussion (hacking) for 10 seconds. Effleurage lightly.

6   Effleurage the top of the shoulder from head to arm. Petrissage for 30 seconds. Perform percussion (hacking) for 10 seconds. Then effleurage in a circular motion.

7   Walk round to the other side of the body, keeping your hand in contact with the body and repeat all the strokes.

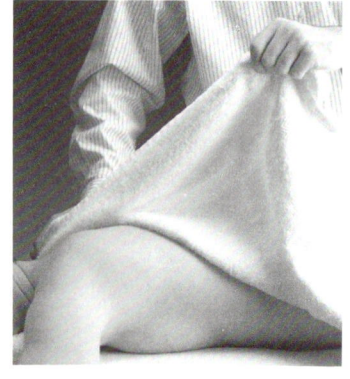

8   Return to position 1. Effleurage as in step 2, this time getting lighter and slower towards the 10th stroke.

9   Cover the back with a towel and ask your partner to breathe deeply three times.

ABOVE STEP 9: COVER YOUR PARTNER WITH A TOWEL AT THE END OF THE MASSAGE TO KEEP HER WARM.

Ask your partner to turn over slowly. Otherwise he or she may make an awkward movement if drowsy, or leap up too fast – and off the couch. Position yourself close to guard against this but don't attempt to lift your partner: instead, develop expertise in removing the pillows from underneath and have them ready to go under the head and thighs as your partner lies back. The pillows are important to enable a partner to relax the limbs and neck and will also prolong the effects of the back massage.

TIP

To prevent straining your own back when giving a back massage, try to keep your knees slightly flexed.

41

LEG MASSAGE

Extraordinary balancers and locomotors, the leg muscles are also adept massagers of their own veins, redirecting spent blood back to the heart against considerable force of gravity. Cardiac patients, formerly ordered to bed and told not to move are now advised to make active leg movements to relieve the strain on their hearts. Commonplace symptoms of cramp and varicosity indicate tiredness in the legs and too much tension above them – treat the legs!

MASSAGE TECHNIQUE

1   Take up position at the feet, facing your partner. Massage the foot of the nearest leg in the same manner as the hand (see p.36), although all strokes can be deeper unless your partner is very sensitive. After squeezing around the big toe, knead down the instep and back again six times.

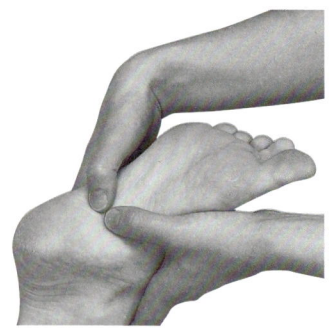 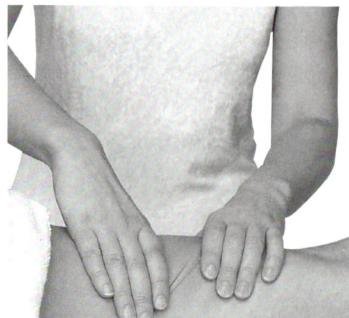

ABOVE STEP 2: STROKES CAN BE DEEP HERE.

ABOVE STEP 7: KNEAD IN A PUSH/PULL ACTION.

2   If your partner has varicose veins omit the kneading and percussion strokes from the following sequence. Bend the leg and stand the foot flat.

3   Effleurage the lower leg with your palm and fingers, following its contours. Stroke from the ankle to the knee, increasing depth, with a stronger up stroke. Do 20 times.

42

4   Knead by squeezing and rolling the calf muscles and press against the outside of the shin with your thumb for 30 seconds. Effleurage deeply five times.

5   Do percussion (hacking) around the lower leg for 15 seconds. Effleurage lightly.

6   Extend the leg over the pillow and move to the side. Effleurage from the ankle to the front of the pelvis 10 times.

7   Place your whole hand across the front and outside of the thigh, thumbs nearest your body. Knead by using close palm contact with fingers together to squeeze the leg in a push/pull action for 30 seconds. Effleurage deeply from knee to pelvis five times.

8   Petrissage on the inner hamstrings of the back of the leg, which can just be felt inside the knee; these and the groin muscles are gently pressed with the fingertips. Begin from the knee and proceed two-thirds of the way along the groin, at which point the muscles separate, and work back down for 30 seconds. Effleurage deeply five times.

9   Do percussion (hacking) all over the thigh for 15 seconds. Effleurage lightly then extend the stroke to the whole leg.

There is an obvious anatomical difference between male and female thighs, with those of men being more muscular and parallel, while women converge at the knee and have greater tension on the outside of the thigh. You may have to go lightly on the front of well-muscled male thighs for comfort and especially light on a female partner's groin, which is sensitive around the time of menstruation.

ARM MASSAGE

The nerves in the body are distributed in such a way that some of those that control the interior organs are directly related to those of the skin. This is particularly true of the chest organs and the skin on the arms. People who experience constriction around the heart often notice peculiar feelings in their arms first because the nervous energy to both areas originates from the same nerve 'root' in the spine. By what is known as 'reflex action' we can send the relaxing benefits of arm massage to the chest. Arm massage is very soothing, especially for those unable to have a full body massage.

MASSAGE TECHNIQUE
1   Position yourself as for hand massage.
2   Perform effleurage by stroking from wrist to elbow 10 times, encircling the arm with both hands.
3   Petrissage softly, squeezing up and down the forearm for 30 seconds. (You are massaging the muscles that move the fingers and you may notice trembling in the hand.)
4   Effleurage deeply five times.

5   To enable you to get to the upper arm comfortably for effleurage, try having your partner hold on to your shoulder, while you bend forward slightly. If this is not satisfactory, the arm can lie flat along the couch, or you can raise it with one hand while the other strokes it. Effleurage from elbow to shoulder 10 times.

6   Knead with both hands close on to the arm, squeezing the muscles away from the bone. Continue up into the shoulder muscle, for 30 seconds. Effleurage deeply five times.

7   Perform percussion (hacking) all around the arm for 15 seconds. Effleurage lightly.

TIP

Be careful when treating the upper arm that you don't press on the 'funny bone', where the ulnar nerve, which supplies the little finger side of the forearm and hand, passes behind the inner side of the elbow joint. It is not at all amusing for your partner as they relax and, from your point of view, if they are holding on to your shoulder at that moment, you may receive an involuntary clip on the ear.

44

CHEST MASSAGE

Women have sensitive breast tissue covering the important arm muscles that lie over the chest wall (the pectoral muscles). Men can also find direct pressure on the chest uncomfortable, so this massage is concerned with drainage points in the circulatory system rather than with the muscles. When these points are very active during menstruation or acute illnesses such as influenza, partners may find chest massage unacceptable; cupping, percussion or frictions over the ribs may, however, relieve congested chests.

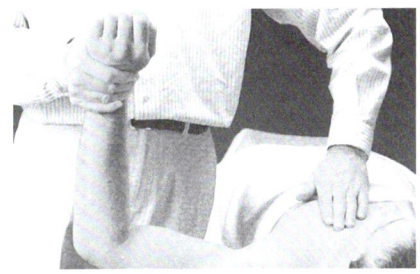

MASSAGE TECHNIQUE

1   Have your partner lie facing upwards; put a small pillow under the shoulders.

2   Effleurage the arm with your inside hand, gliding along the chest just beneath the collarbone and on to the breastbone. Make the return stroke to the armpit slightly stronger. Repeat four times.

3   Walk your fingertips or knuckles from the breastbone to the armpit, in this direction only. With male partners you may use the heel of the hand as well as the fingers. Repeat four times. Effleurage as at 2.

45

4   Support the arm and move it gently around the shoulder, lightly stretching it away from the body to release tension in the chest muscles.

5   After massaging both sides of the chest, ask your partner to breathe deeply while you compress their rib cage on exhalation. Place your hands flat against the outsides of the chest and squeeze gently, releasing to allow a deeper breath in.

TIP

You can combine chest massage with massage of the back by having your partner lie on their side. It is then possible to treat half of the back with the shoulders and rib cage; try the cupping percussion to help with congestion inside the chest.

ABDOMINAL MASSAGE

We are cautions about being touched around the abdomen, perhaps because it contains our vital organs and seems a very intimate part of our body, or perhaps it just feels relatively unprotected. The abdomen is indeed a highly nervous area and, combined with these other considerations, it is not surprising that some partners find this massage unbearably ticklish. You might find that you are creating more tension than relaxation by working in this area, but persevere because it is a very beneficial massage. Experiment by practising on your own abdomen to develop an acceptable touch for your partner.

MASSAGE TECHNIQUE

1   Stand to the side of your partner close to the couch. Effleurage around the abdomen 10 times in a clockwise direction. Stroke gently but not too lightly, otherwise you will stimulate reflexes in the abdomen.

2   Next use a combined effleurage/pressure stroke that relaxes the waist muscles. Cross your arms and place your palms against and slightly underneath the waist; squeeze and lift up the waist, then let the body slip between the hand as you pass across the abdomen. Fold your arms alternately one above the other and repeat six times. Effleurage.

3   Knead the centre of the abdomen with your fingers stretched from the thumbs, up and down from the ribs to the front of the pelvis six times. (Go more lightly as you near the bladder, which is in the lower abdomen.) Effleurage.

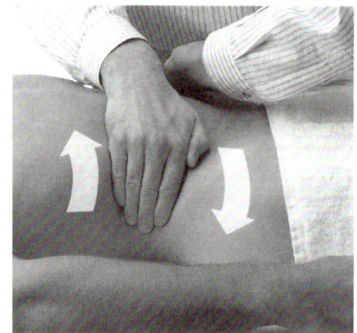

4   Use the edge and the palm of your hands alternately to make firm waves in a

ABOVE STEP 2: AVOID PRESSING DOWN AS YOU PERFORM THE RETURN STROKE HERE..

46

scooping motion from the lower to the upper abdomen 20 times. This stroke encourages the lower back muscles to relax and tips the pelvis backwards; the abdominal contents, which are dragged down by gravity, are repositioned and abdominal congestion is relieved. Effleurage.

5   Repeat crossovers and effleurage as before 10 times.

TIP

Abdominal massage is recommended as an excellent self-massage. Women may find the scooping (step 4) particularly helpful for menstrual pains when combined with low back massage. Massaging the abdomen can also help low spirits when life feels like a burden, by stimulating the nerve endings in the abdominal plexus, and raising energy.

47

NECK MASSAGE (LYING DOWN)

Our neck keeps our head high but it is also an important bridge between the brain and the rest of the body. Considering the extreme tensions from which the neck can suffer, it is remarkable that communications are so good. This is because the neck is a very flexible and resilient structure – as long as its muscles are sufficiently relaxed. Anxieties and worries increase the neck's tension and our shoulders tend to rise as problems mount.

MASSAGE TECHNIQUE

1   Have your partner lie facing upwards, and take up position at the head. Perform all the movements in this massage extremely slowly, and explain to your partner clearly what you intend to do.

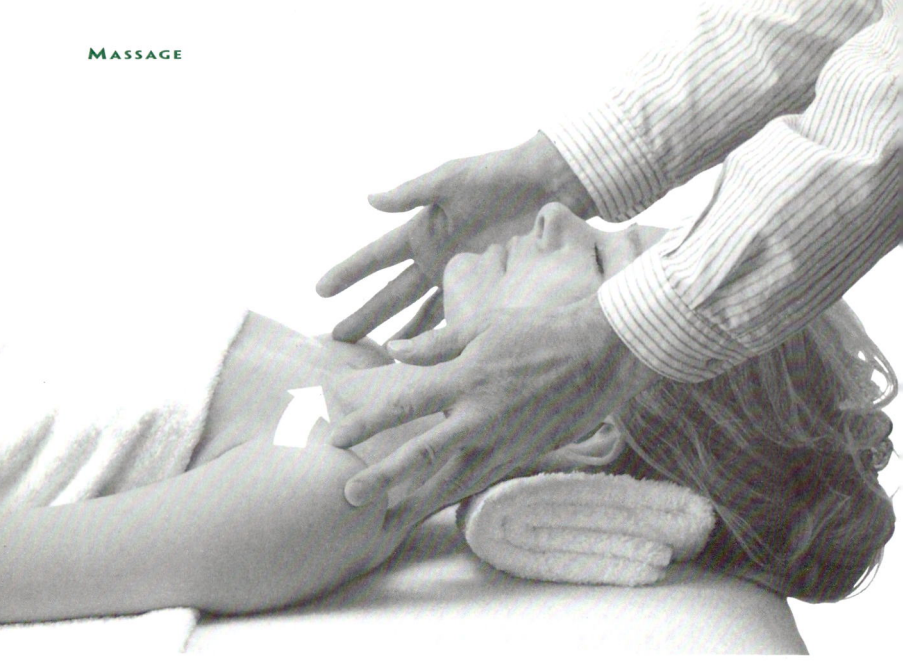

ABOVE MAKE SURE THAT YOUR PARTNER'S HEAD IS WELL SUPPORTED ON A ROLLED-UP TOWEL BEFORE BEGINNING THE NECK MASSAGE.

2   Roll the head gently to the left side, like a ball, not raising it. Use your right hand to effleurage evenly up and down the neck on to the shoulder 10 times. Roll the head to the other side and repeat.

3   Returning the head to the left side, place your fingers under the neck and your thumb along its side. Knead gently by pushing and releasing the hand against the neck. Avoid pressing directly with the thumb. Do this for 30 seconds and then repeat on the other side of the neck.

4   Place the head in the central position. Using both hands, repeat the squeezing stroke from the base of the skull up and down the back of the neck.

5   Next, following the sequence below, perform some safe stretches on your partner. You will feel a 'give' while stretching the neck muscles that is due to the loosening effect of prior kneading.

Providing you keep the movements slow, your partner will always be in control of the stretch. However, do not stretch middle-aged partners, who may be losing suppleness, without close supervision.

a   Roll the head to the right with your left hand, then, crossing your forearms, place your right hand against the left shoulder. Ask your partner to take a long inhalation. As he or she exhales, slowly and evenly stretch the head towards the right shoulder, for the duration of the out-breath. If the chin goes well towards the shoulder, the stretch is quite sufficient. Very slowly roll the head to the other side and repeat.

b   Support the head in both hands and stretch forwards. The chin may almost touch the chest. Use the same breathing rhythm as for the previous stretch.

c   Hold the whole head firmly but comfortably. As your partner exhales, draw the head away from the body. This may seem very adventurous but is in fact a simple movement! The stretch relies on the stronger downward force exerted by the exhalation rather than on your 'pull', so there is less actual force used than in the previous stretches.

6   Effleurage lightly around the head, neck and shoulders. You may like to improvise a face massage as your partner relaxes.

NECK MASSAGE (SEATED)

When someone has an established arthritic condition that has affected the wrists or hands, it may also have damaged the stability of the joints of the neck; in this case you can offer the following, very gentle, version of neck massage with your partner sitting upright. This has the advantage that pressure from tensions are easily drawn downwards and the posture of the neck and head improved. This can be a very spontaneous massage, done almost anywhere, and has converted many sceptics to the pleasure of whole body treatments.

MASSAGE TECHNIQUE

1   Standing behind, eff-
leurage from the sides
of the head down the
neck and over the
shoulders to the upper
arms. Repeat six times.

2   Perform tight petri-
ssage on the ridge
of the shoulders. Use
the thumbs, resting
the fingers over the
shoulders, moving from
the centre to the
outside edges for 30
seconds. Effleurage as before.

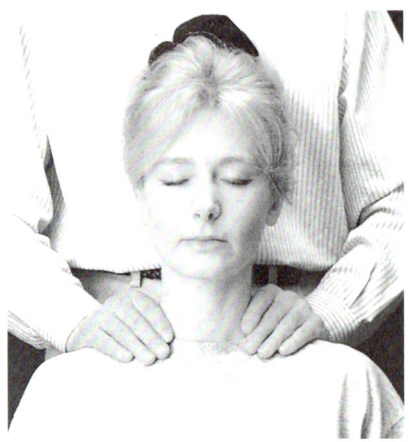

ABOVE NECK MASSAGE GIVEN IN THIS POSITION ENSURES THAT PRESSURE FROM TENSION IS EASILY DRAWN DOWNWARD.

50

3   Hold your partner's forehead in the palm of your right hand and pinch up and down the back of the neck with your left hand for 30 seconds. Repeat, changing your hands around. Perform effleurage as before.

4   Allow the head to rest back against your abdomen. Effleurage from the forehead to the temples, and from the chin to the temples, six times.

5   Petrissage, using the fingertips to circle lightly over the face (very gently near the eyes) for 30 seconds. Effleurage as before.

6   Use percussion (tapotement), with your fingertips drumming all over the face for 15 seconds. Effleurage.

7   Replace the head in the upright position and, still supporting it with one hand, effleurage one side six times from the head through the neck and shoulders to the upper arm. Repeat on the other side.

8   Ask your partner to support fully his or her neck, and repeat effleurage with both hands, six times, each stroke becoming lighter and lighter.

AFTERCARE

Having finished the massage, cover your partner with a towel and keep him or her warm so as to continue the sense of being cared for. A massaged partner might be drowsy or asleep or may want to talk; you should be available for his or her time of transition back to 'normality' but it may be that you feel the need to withdraw. Professionals recognize this possibility by giving a 50-minute massage in an hour's treatment so as to allow a few minutes for a satisfactory ending. In a busy practice it is easy to forget how valuable this time can be for both so it is a habit you can adopt from the outset.

SPECIAL MASSAGES

After completing the strokes of a treatment, you can increase your partner's sense of relaxation by a technique known as 'mobilizing'. This involves moving each joint slowly through its natural range of movement, with co-operation but not assistance from your partner. Simply allowing someone else to move our body is not easy and, even when apparently willing, partners are often unable to relax and let go completely. This is an indication of how tensions sometimes represent an investment of energy that can get locked up in the body. By patiently waiting and moving sensitively, rather than forcing, you will eventually be able to move their body with lessening resistance.

MOBILIZE THE LIMBS

The arm and leg joints are designed to move freely, and they have lubricating fluids to ensure smoothness. Movement normally occurs from muscles pulling across the joint, and when we mobilize our partner our hands take the place of their muscles.

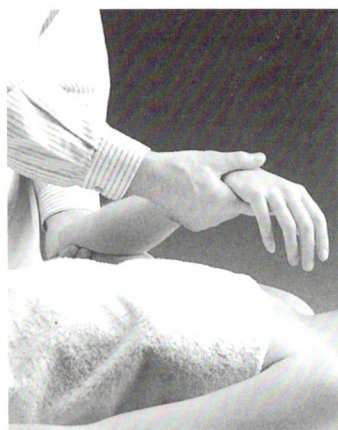

ABOVE THE PASSIVE MOVEMENTS CREATE PLEASANT
SENSATIONS SIMILAR TO THOSE OF GENTLE SWIMMING.

For maximum benefit you should move the joints the way they seem to want to go and just a little further. Support the elbow in your palm and hold your partner's hand in the other. Slowly bend the elbow, pausing when you feel your partner 'helping', until it is fully flexed and then extend it straight. Repeat until the elbow joint opens and closes with ease. Notice that the elbow flexes with the palm turned up or down, and mobilize in both directions.

MOBILIZE THE SHOULDERS

52

Anxiety and monotonous posture severely reduce what should be 360° mobility of the shoulder. Check your partner's shoulder mobility: for example, can he or she swing the right arm over the head, take the left arm behind the back and, bending the elbow, touch the fingers? If not, the following movement will be beneficial.

1 Ask your partner to lie sideways, with a pillow under the head and the top leg bending forwards for steadiness.

2 Lightly massage the arm and side of the neck.

3 Thread your arm through theirs, supporting its weight. Hold the shoulder with both your hands.

4 Move the shoulder up and down, then forwards and backwards. As your partner relaxes and the arm feels

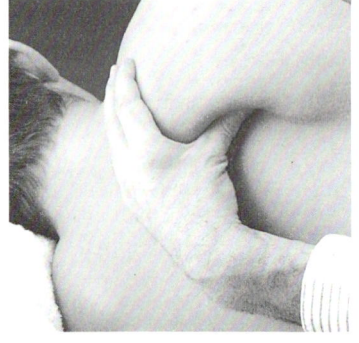

ABOVE STEP 4: PRESS THE THUMBS DEEPLY ALONG THE EDGE OF THE SHOULDER BONE.

heavier, begin a circular movement. If you can get your fingertips under the shoulder-blade, this will release more tension.

5   Replace the arm, and effleurage before asking your partner to turn over slowly. Repeat the movements to the other side.

Many people find this a soporific treatment; if your partner falls asleep by the end of the massage to the second shoulder, he or she probably needs to. Cover your partner over and stay close by.

MOBILIZE THE HIP

Stiffness in the hip is accompanied by increased buttock tension on the affected side, which can be observed with your partner facing downwards. This treatment also helps with pains in the leg that have origins in the lower back; for example, the unpleasant sensation radiating down the back of the leg, known as sciatica, when the pressure affects the great sciatic nerve.

53

1   Ask your partner to lie face down. Place a small pillow under the abdomen and a large pillow under the feet. Check the tension in the buttocks.

2   Put one hand flat against the upper thigh while slowly raising and lowering the foot. When there is a problem in the hip, the knee joint will not move easily.

3   Push hard on to the thigh with your palm as you flex the knee, then lower the foot slowly, releasing the pressure as the foot touches the pillow.

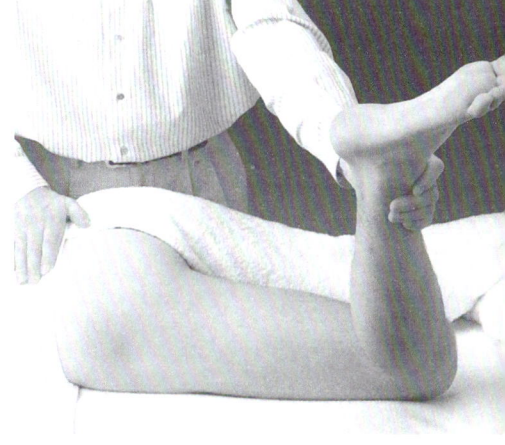

ABOVE IF THERE IS ANY PROBLEM IN THE HIP, YOU'LL FIND THAT THE KNEE JOINT WILL FEEL A BIT INFLEXIBLE.

4   Repeat three times. Check for reduced tension in the buttock, and treat both legs until equally relaxed. (For one-sided tension, place a pillow under the pelvic bone on the opposite side.)

MOBILIZE THE NECK

The joints of the neck have a wide range of movement, unlike the rest of the spine which has to accommodate and support the chest and pelvis.

However, the graceful curves of the neck are easily forfeited to fixed occupational postures, and this mobilization is an attempt to remind us of the neck's full potential.

1   Ask your partner to lie towards the top of the couch so that the head and neck extends beyond the end of the couch, and support the head with your hands. This is very testing of the trust between you; if the head should slip from your hands, your partner would probably recover control but their neck muscles might never forgive you.

   (For the reassurance of both parties, you may place a smaller table under the head so the distance below is less but still enough to allow movement. Before you begin the mobilization, read through the whole text, then give your complete attention to the movements.)

2   Very slowly move the head up and down and from side to side. If you are successful, you will feel the head increasingly heavy as the neck relaxes.

3   Lower the head a little and hold it quite still. Rotate it to each side and while it is fully turned, lower it a little further. This is the most helpful movement so don't rush it.

4   Repeat all the movements, checking that your partner still feels comfortable. You may be able to tell that the neck muscles are more relaxed this time. Finish by supporting the head to allow recovery back down on to the couch. Place the head on a small pillow and ask your partner to breathe deeply.

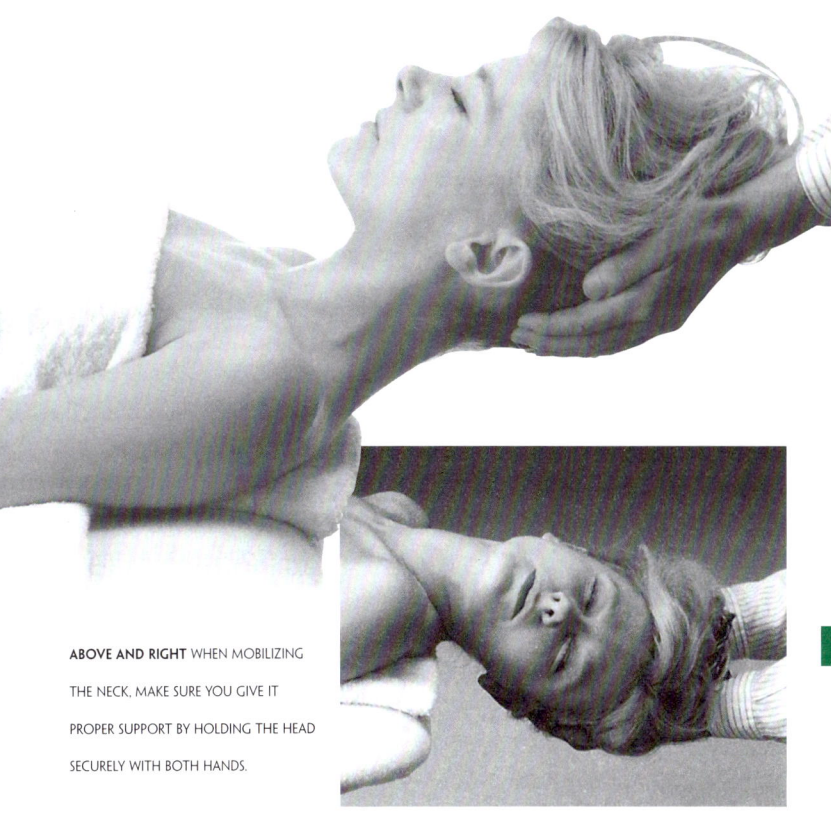

ABOVE AND RIGHT WHEN MOBILIZING THE NECK, MAKE SURE YOU GIVE IT PROPER SUPPORT BY HOLDING THE HEAD SECURELY WITH BOTH HANDS.

Mobilizations can be very helpful after injury or illness to bring confidence back to movements. After a period of immobility, even everyday movements can be painful, whereas your mobilizations should be painless. Your partner may feel disoriented after giving you responsibility for their movements, so be aware of possible unsteadiness as they get up, and caution them to move slowly at first.

Gain experience of applying the mobilizations on your fittest partners, who can join you in a spirit of investigation! If you consider a deeper movement might be of special help to someone, double check with them first for contra-indications. It is unlikely that you could cause harm but you may find all your earlier relaxing work undone if a partner is unprepared for deeper massage.

REVIEW YOUR PROGRESS

Before going on to look at the specific applications of massage, let's review your practice so far:

ARE YOU ENJOYING THE MASSAGE
AS MUCH AS YOUR PARTNERS APPEAR TO BE?

So that your energy keeps pace with your enthusiasm, don't spend much more than an hour treating someone. Too long a session can become debilitating for you and your partner and, if you increase the number of your treatments, you won't be able to give everyone a very long session.

ARE YOU LEARNING MORE ABOUT THE BODY?

During even the briefest treatment your partner is offering you a lesson and an opportunity to understand how the body works. Without making your partner feel like a 'specimen', adapt your treatment plan according to any changes in their condition.

ARE YOU AWARE OF ANY EMOTIONAL STRAIN
CONNECTED WITH GIVING MASSAGES?

Even if you intend to steer clear of your partner's life-problems, there may be occasions when your own mood makes you vulnerable to another's distress. How will you handle this? If your treatments seem to be going well you may not have connected fluctuations in your own emotions with the act of giving massage. Tiredness can be as much a sign of this kind of strain as over-exertion, and you should realize that your emotional muscles need as much conditioning as those that you use to perform massage. Professionals learn to dissociate themselves from one person's problems to the next, through an appointment system that encourages exclusive concentration on the specific problem at hand. In a more casual atmosphere, it may still help you to follow other formal procedures such as thorough hand-washing, or making a few notes on your reactions to a session. In the longer term, it is advisable not to 'carry' your partner's emotional material even when it may feel manageable; partners who seem to need more out of massage than you are able to give should be referred on to experienced practitioners.

IS YOUR PRACTICE GROWING?

The more massage you give and the more experienced you become, the clearer it will become which part of the body or aspect of the strokes you are naturally drawn towards. Partners often feel in need of particular attention, which is acknowledged, even though we recognize the necessity of treating the whole body. Make it known to partners that you are developing an interest in treating common sites of tension. In certain situations, this may be the only route to access deeper but treatable problems that general massages fail to relieve.

57

RIGHT AS YOUR SKILL AND CONFIDENCE DEVELOP,
YOUR SENSITIVITY TO YOUR EACH INDIVIDUAL'S
PARTICULAR NEEDS WILL INCREASE.

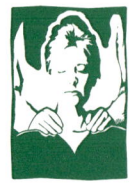

WHAT MASSAGE DOES

O nce you have some experience of massage, both you and your partner will have begun to realize why it has such a deserved reputation as a therapy. The permission we give others to massage us is not given lightly, however, and passively submitting to being touched is not the same as allowing ourselves to be moved; it is the establishment of trust and co-operation that allows the strokes of massage to be truly beneficial to the mind and body.

PHYSICAL AND EMOTIONAL BENEFITS

The many benefits of massage can be measured and have been well researched by practitioners. This is made easy because of the persuasiveness of the muscles throughout the body, and because their skillful manipulation has such a profound effect on it: they assist the circulation in the blood and lymphatic vessels, stimulate the organs of digestion and elimination and improve the performance of the lungs and skin. As the muscles themselves improve in tone, so do the nerves that supply them to the spinal cord and back to the brain. The nerves provide the stimulus for movement and feeling and are extremely sensitive and alert to the atmosphere inside and outside the body.

It is not easy to evaluate massage psychologically except that most people agree it is a potentially pleasurable experience.

CASE STUDY: TREATING HIGH BLOOD PRESSURE

An older adult who reported a sudden onset of 'dizziness' was seen by her doctor who diagnosed high blood pressure. Although the patient had been the same weight over many years the treatment prescribed was to lose weight quickly by dieting.

After no change in weight or blood pressure, a sympathetic friend made arrangements for massage treatments. The initial session revealed severe tension in her neck and shoulders. During the session, the patient hinted at an emotional crisis involving the reappearance of another person in her life and the strain it was causing. It was a painful but just bearable situation to which the restrictive diet for her weight problem was felt as a further affliction. When reassurance was given that raised blood pressure was not unnatural where there was emotional strain, the shoulders became much more massageable.

As massage treatments continued and a near normal diet resumed, the situation showed some signs of being resolved and her blood pressure dropped. The sessions were punctuated by considerable distress, however, when the patient spoke of the background to the crisis. Eventually she was able to speak the unsaid to her friend and life gradually became more peaceful.

Perhaps this could be considered a straightforward case except that the patient was as much concerned with her reaction to the crisis as to its cause. What was massage able to offer this person?

59

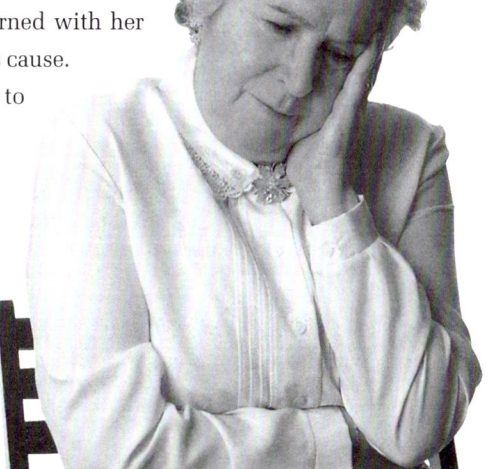

RIGHT AS MASSAGE IS A HOLISTIC THERAPY IT CAN HELP TO TREAT EMOTIONAL ISSUES AS WELL AS PHYSICAL PROBLEMS.

HOW THE MASSAGE WORKED

1   Sometimes a medical diagnosis can be a welcome distraction from a problem, but here it only emphasized an aspect of the problem and in a punitive way. The massage highlighted the tension in the neck and shoulders as being connected with emotional pressure, and thus the alarm of the original diagnosis (which itself was contributing to the emotional strain) was minimized.

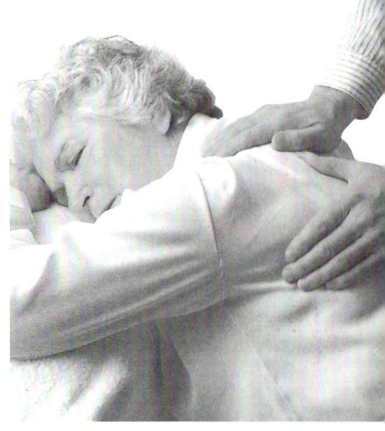

ABOVE THE ACT OF MASSAGE IS EMOTIONALLY SUPPORTIVE.

2   The treatment of the shoulders and arms allowed freer circulation between the extremities and the chest (which tends to become restricted with unhappiness or anger). Nervous controls shared by the chest and arms were also influenced, so that deeper breathing, a reliever of pressure, was induced.

3   The treatments enabled the person to use the supportive atmosphere of the massage treatment to express herself. This is quite different from a response in conversation or analysis in that it was accepted that the problem had become physically manifested in the body. Her dialogue with the practitioner was able to move between the verbal and the muscular according to her feelings; where words failed, focus returned to the muscles, and when tension was greatest, words came.

TENSION AND POSTURE

The tensions created by fear can affect our posture. Sometimes we respond to unsolvable problems by pushing our chin forward, pulling our arms tight against our sides, or twisting our pelvis in an attempt to draw away. In similar situations animals pretend to grow

60

RELEASING FEAR AND NEGATIVE EMOTION

Fear, often from past experience, influences our emotional life. When we are initially frightened, our body sets up special safeguards that are entirely defensive. Unless we have become stiff with fright, we are usually being prepared for almost heroic action; when circumstances frustrate activity, acute tension is produced. A common response is to react with a displacing response, such as eating. In one sense this is curious, since we have little power of digestion when afraid; undigested foods are not absorbed but give rise to substances that are circulated around the body and can ultimately lead to the tensing of muscles and stiffening of joints characteristic of rigid fear. In the short term a sense of stiffness and unease brings a genuine feeling of distress, as we enter a vicious cycle where the original problem is easily obscured. From a dietary point of view the option to eat may be a variation on primitive chewing, to which chewing gum and smoking may be heirs.

If what we are seeking from eating is reassurance, the safe touch of massage may provide the answer. The physical contact needs to be genuine rather than expert, though for some people it takes time to get used to having someone else handle their stress. The massager is then in a position to shift our awareness from frustration or bewilderment to a more grounded experience of how our body is coping with the situation.

in size, but humans usually end up diminished. Unreleased tension causes shortening of the spine, which begins to show in an expanded abdomen, flattening of the feet, and a backward tilt of the head. As well as relieving this tension, massage is able to remould our posture.

Improved posture releases us from a subtle cycle of strain. If a taller person stoops, does this make them appear more or less threatening

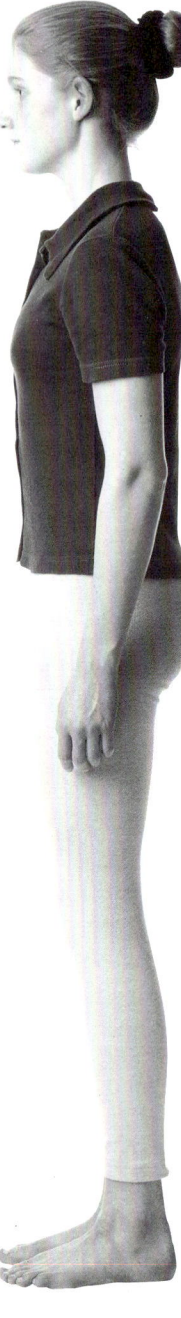

to people smaller than themselves? When we draw back our pelvis when others come near, do we realize this gives the impression that we are about to fall towards them? Because we are using more effort to maintain such a posture, we may convince our friends that we are relaxed, but sooner or later it begins to hurt. Massagers are immediately aware of inconsistent posture, and their treatments aim to challenge the tension without removing it prematurely. It is as if we say to ourselves: 'I feel anxious so I'll arch my back' but forget that after a short time an arching back also creates anxiety. It would be better to discover this with the help of massage than to develop a chronic problem that has to be corrected by more drastic means.

The movements of massage create a sense of space within our posture and give us the chance to reassess our reactions to problems in life. They offer a way to poise amidst the many stresses that surround us, allowing a more constructive use of our muscles.

Your development in massage will be enhanced by combining the confidence that comes from knowledge with your natural ability to treat. Everything you discover about how massage benefits an injury or illness will be an inspiration in your work to raise healthy bodies to an even healthier level.

LEFT BAD POSTURE, OFTEN CAUSED BY PHYSICAL OR EMOTIONAL TENSION, CAN BE RECTIFIED BY REGULAR MASSAGE TREATMENTS.

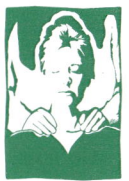

MASSAGE TREATMENTS

CHAPTER SEVEN

A variety of massage techniques is used today, ranging from aromatherapy, which uses essential plant oils, through to polarity therapy, which uses positive energy to heal emotional problems. Usually, these techniques are treatments whose applications have consistently improved a condition or relieved a problem where general treatments have failed. They are often mysterious, glamourous or personalized, and are available on very expensive courses. In this chapter I outline several very useful techniques, and explain the particular benefits of each.

AROMATHERAPY

Massage using oil that has been blended with the essence of a plant is known as aromatherapy. The essences themselves are a little oily, very fragrant, and

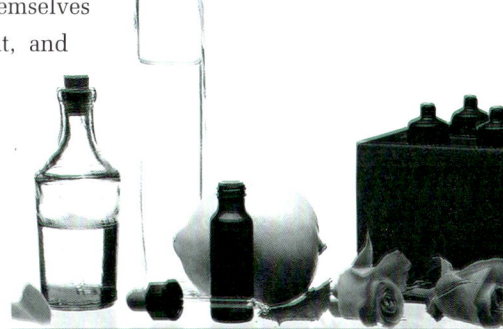

RIGHT EACH OIL HAS A DIFFERENT EFFECT ON THE MIND AND BODY. FOR EXAMPLE, SOME ARE CALMING AND SOME INVIGORATING.

usually too concentrated to be used undiluted. They are extracted by a variety of methods according to whether the fruit, leaf or stem of the plant is used.

Vast amounts of raw materials are required to produce even a small amount of essential oil, and their harvesting and lengthy production make them expensive.

Essential oils have been used therapeutically since Biblical times. The discovery of their chemical composition in recent years has brought about an increasing use of synthetic scents, but these have become the perfumes of the cosmetics industry. Though incomparable, the new essences were far cheaper to produce and their high alcohol content meant they could be kept indefinitely. The current trend back towards more natural products has fortunately led to a revival in demand for true essential oils, and their original role is being rediscovered.

Research has shown that essential oils possess the medicinal properties associated with herbs, are antiseptic and capable of adjusting a person's mood via the olfactory nerves. Although the oils are highly concentrated, they are without side-effects if used properly, although a person's reaction to treatment may sometimes be very emotional.

Aromatherapy massages are given in part rather than a whole body treatment, with periods of calm effleurage to allow a partner to appreciate the fragrance of the oil.

AROMATHERAPY FOR THE FACE

OIL – LEMONGRASS

1   Stand or sit at your partner's head within easy reach of the face. A towel or head band can be used to clear away the hair.

2   Place a few drops of blended oil on your hand and spread it lightly on to the face. Effleurage the face from the chin to the temples and across the forehead 10 times.

3   Make circular strokes with your fingertips on the cheeks for 10 seconds. Effleurage towards the ears.

4   Do similar strokes along the jaw line to its hinges beside the ears. Reverse and, reaching the chin, continue around the mouth, moving the lips but without opening the mouth. Repeat six times. Effleurage.

5   Stroke the rims of the eye sockets with one finger three times. Make the strokes firmer on the upper rim.

6   Look for tension lines on the forehead – horizontal, vertical or both – and rub at right angles for 10 seconds. Effleurage deeply upwards and outwards.

7   Hold the ear lobes and pull gently down and away from the head three times.

8   Percuss the whole face with tapotement – fingertips drumming – avoiding the eyes.

9   Effleurage the face from the chin to the temples and across the forehead 10 times. The finishing strokes should be very light.

10 Comb through the hair with your fingers, lightly scratching the scalp. Take good handfuls of hair and squeeze or pull until the scalp stretches three times.

65

You will not be able to return to stroke the face after hair pulling, so complete the treatment by effleuraging the shoulders.

BELOW USE A HEADBAND OR TOWEL TO HOLD THE HAIR BACK. POUR JUST A FEW DROP OF THE BLENDED OIL INTO THE PALM OF YOUR HAND.

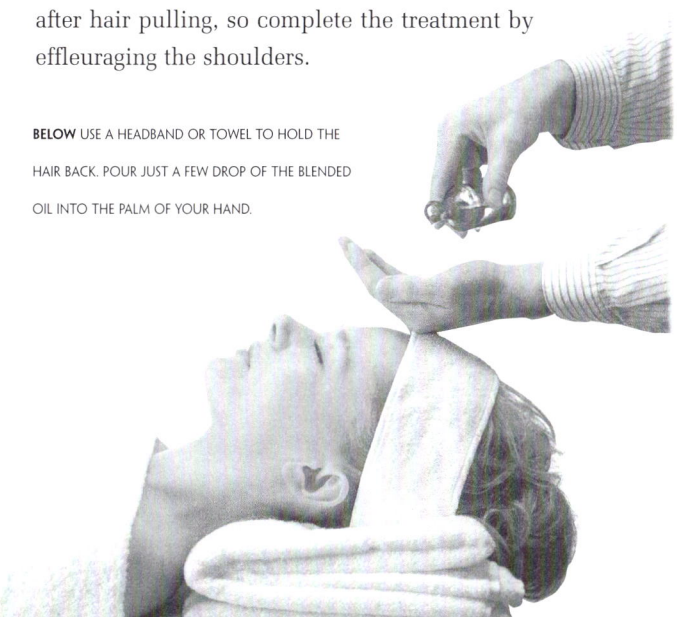

OUR TIRED FACES

Although we strive to maintain the hygiene of our face, from a massager's point of view it really is a neglected area of the body. Our fixed expressions keep the muscles of the face in tension over long periods, and the combination of polluted city-life and the effects of air-conditioning are very damaging to the skin. Neck tension further adds to the pressures that build up, especially around our eyes, impeding their circulation and drainage.

An aromatherapy facial massage is a wonderful way to relieve facial tension.

AROMATHERAPY FOR THE BACK

This is an excellent treatment for relieving back stiffness and pain after exertion.

66

OIL – SAGE

1   Before applying the oil, friction the whole back with palms and fingertips to increase circulation to the skin.
2   Stand at the head of your partner. Pour a teaspoonful of oil into your hands and apply to the whole back. (You may need more later according to the skin type.)
3   Perform reverse effleurage, repeating 10 times, stroking down the centre of the back. Return via the waist and sides of the chest to the armpit.
4   Using your fingertips, 'rake' all over the back.

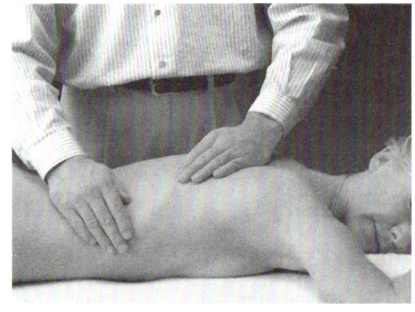

ABOVE STEP 1: START BY RUNNING YOUR PALMS AND FINGERTIPS OVER THE BACK TO INCREASE CIRCULATION.

5   Use the edge of your hands or knuckles to glide over the back at different angles.

6   Snatch at the skin from the spine to the edge of the chest and from the shoulders to the pelvis, concentrating around the shoulders. Effleurage deeply.

7   Twist the skin into an 'S' shape using your thumbs.

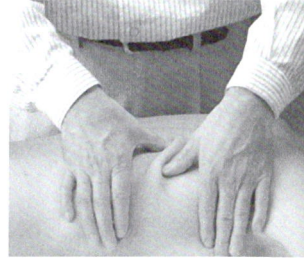

8   Pick up the skin and roll it between your thumbs and fingers from the upper to lower back and to the sides of the chest.

9   Repeat reverse effleurage, giving a deep stretch to the lower back, and on return draw the shoulders wide.

ABOVE STEP 7: USING YOUR

10 Cover your partner and keep him or her warm. Allow extra time for your partner to recover from an aromatherapy treatment.

THUMBS, TWIST THE SKIN

WITHOUT PINCHING IT.

Don't try to knead the muscles of the back using oil because you won't have enough control. Instead, direct your strokes to the skin, toning it and increasing the circulation to the muscles underneath. When your partner is feeling tender from emotion or too much exertion, this skin-deep technique is more acceptable and painless, while still conditioning the muscles underneath.

HYDROTHERAPY (WATER THERAPY)

Hydrotherapy is used in conjunction with massage to relieve common problems. The effect of water on the body can relieve pain, improve circulation and act as a tonic. Animals practise a form of hydrotherapy by licking their wounds and by immersing themselves in streams when injured. Father Kneipp, a 19th century priest and healer, pioneered the use of hydrotherapy in his Bavarian clinic, and became famous for successfully treating many human disorders.

HOW HYDROTHERAPY WORKS

The benefits of water therapy come from the reaction of our warm-blooded bodies; brief applications of water of different temperatures on the skin usually have an opposite effect; cold water acts tonically on the body and is usually preferred to hot, but how cold depends on the individual's make-up. Slender people require cold only slightly beneath blood temperature, whereas substantial bodies react better to an extreme. Our alarm at the prospect of coming into contact with chilly water is based on the expectation of a long immersion. However, our bodies tolerate cold much more readily than too much heat, as babies and those who recover from freezing conditions remind us; overheating is much more dangerous for our systems. Hot treatments, which should be applied gradually, are used to soothe and relax and are especially effective on the back of the body.

HYDROTHERAPY FOR MUSCLE SPASM OF THE CALF

It is difficult to relax the great tension of a muscle spasm due to the chemical and nervous conditions within the muscle at that time, which make it hypersensitive. Even if we can get a moderate pressure on to the affected part, it may still be insufficient. We could try more pressure and attempt to replace the first pain by a greater pain – like biting on a toothache – but we may injure ourselves more. The following method is a much safer way of bringing relief:

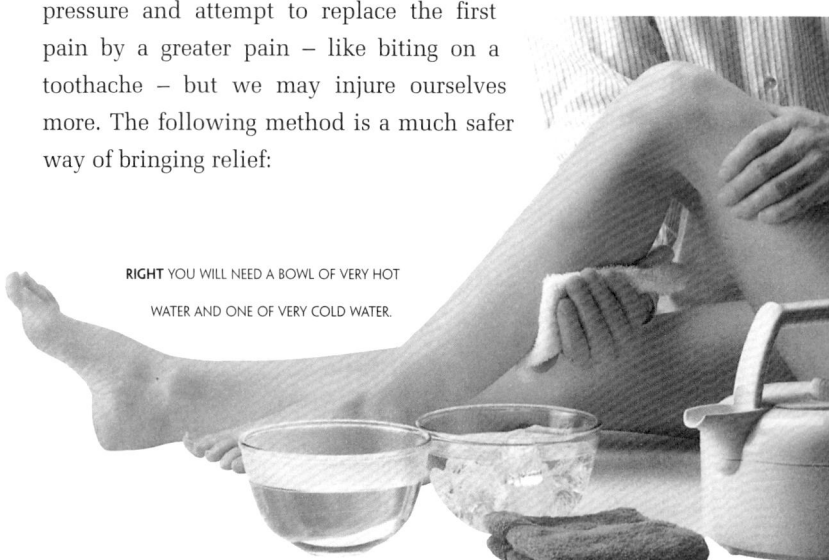

RIGHT YOU WILL NEED A BOWL OF VERY HOT WATER AND ONE OF VERY COLD WATER.

1   Have one bowl of very hot water and one of cold. Keep a hot kettle and a bag of ice nearby to 'top-up'. Soak a face flannel in each; apply the wrung out hot cloth for 30 seconds, then the cold for 30 seconds. Repeat six times, re-soaking the cloth between applications. (After the initial hot and cold, the temperature will feel less extreme and you can add from the kettle and ice bag after three times.)

2   Massage the muscle for three minutes, using deep effleurage. Cover and keep warm.

This hydrotherapy works well on the limbs and neck; trunk muscles, especially on the back, respond better to short, hot immersions in a bath: 3–5 minutes before and after the massage.

HYDROTHERAPY FOR VARICOSE VEINS

The venous blood, returning to the heart near the surface of the body in soft-walled vessels, can suffer impediments. The blood in the legs has the added resistance of gravity to overcome, and when pressures are great in the abdomen, or during pregnancy, the veins stretch and the blood 'queues' rather than flows – the veins swell and the legs ache.

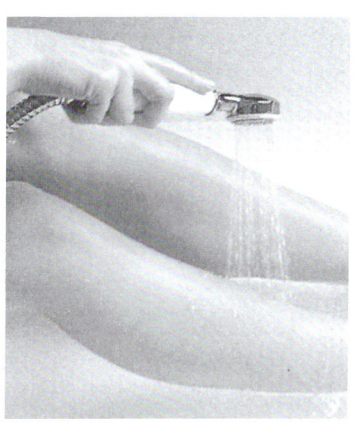

ABOVE SPRAY THE COLD WATER FROM ANKLE TO KNEE.

This technique provides a helpful effleurage, which does not pressurize a painful vein.

1   Sit in a warm bath with your legs out of the water. Use a cold hand shower (or have a friend pour cold water) from the ankle to the knee but not back down, at least 12 times.

2   Dry the body but only wrap the legs in the towel. Rest with pillows under the lower legs, knees bent for 10 minutes.

3   Give back and abdominal massage to relieve the strain on varicose veins.

OSTEOPATHY

Osteopathy is a form of manipulative treatment, conceived in the 19th century by Andrew Taylor-Still in Kansas, USA. Taylor-Still was a compassionate observer of the structure of bodies and he contended that our skeletal posture strongly influences the functioning of the other systems, particularly the nerves. Osteopathic techniques concentrate on releasing 'lesions', areas of abnormal tension, especially around the spinal column. Osteopaths have a rigorous training to become specialists in muscle, joint and bone disorders. The technique has the reputation for equally vigorous application, but in recent years the popular image of back-cracking has given way to a more gentle style.

70

OSTEOPATHY FOR THE HIP JOINT

The technique described is of the milder approach and relies on the co-operation of your partner. It can be used on any of the limb joints. It is particularly useful after an

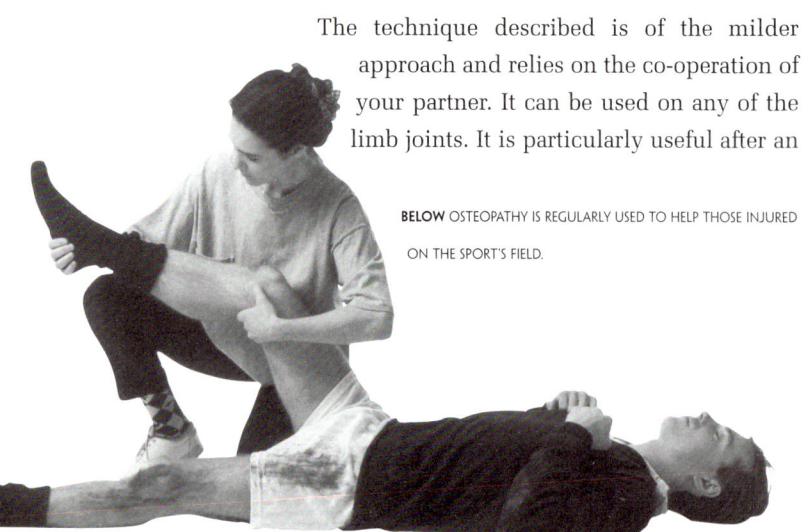

BELOW OSTEOPATHY IS REGULARLY USED TO HELP THOSE INJURED ON THE SPORT'S FIELD.

injury has healed leaving stiffness; when a job or recreation results in one side of the body becoming lighter than the other; or as a relaxing movement after a whole body massage.

1   Have your partner lie flat on his or her back. Fold one knee as close as possible up to the chest. Repeat with the other leg and compare the flexion at the hip.

2   After relaxing both legs down, fold the stiffer leg up and gently press it as far as you can towards the chest. Pause.

3   Ask your partner to push steadily against your pressure, while you resist equally so that you counteract their effort. Hold this position for five seconds.

4   Ask your partner to relax slowly. As their pressure decreases, slowly follow through, pressing their leg closer to the chest. Lean against the leg rather than pushing with your hands, and expect the joint to release a little.

5   Re-starting from this improved position, repeat the technique twice more. It should be painless and your partner will be surprised at how much they can give. You are not forcing the hip but rather guiding the leg into space created by releasing the hip's antagonistic muscles.

71

TIP

If your partner has a rheumatic condition of their joint, you may not achieve much improvement in position and they will feel pain on pressure. If you have their confidence, however, you can do the technique without 'following through', which will help relax the joint and perhaps relieve the pain of stiffness. If, however, they have had a hip joint replacement, beware! Forced flexions of an artificial joint can result in dislocation. Simply supporting the leg, with knee flexed, while your partner moves will help loosen up the muscles safely.

POLARITY THERAPY

Randolph Stone (1890–1983), an Austrian who lived in the USA and India, is accredited as the father of polarity therapy, which he described as a blending of oriental techniques. Polarity therapy is a subtle technique, which regards the body as an energy system, with "positive" and "negative" aspects:

- +   at the head;
- −   at the feet;
- +   to the front;
- −   to the back.

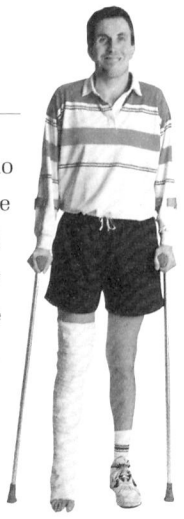

ABOVE POLARITY THERAPY CAN BE HELPFUL FOR INACCESSIBLE INJURIES.

The therapist places a polarizing hand (+ = right) over a partner's uncomfortable area and, using little or no contact, produces a balancing effect.

WHEN TO USE POLARITY THERAPY

Polarity is especially useful when someone's muscles are so tense as to make massage difficult, or when they are impossible to touch, for instance, if they are in a plaster cast. It is also particularly concerned with the physical discomforts that arise with psychological problems. The use of the technique in chronic tension can have a strong emotional effect on partners. I used the technique on someone who had been trying various treatments over some years. After 10 minutes of polarity (his eyes were closed and he was unable to see where my hands were positioned), he spoke of unlocking sensations in his head. 'I don't know what you were doing, but I couldn't take much more of that !' Do not be surprised at your partner's responses that can accompany release of tension: sighing, coughing, laughing or crying. Be sure you feel able to accept spontaneous emotional expression before you decide to use polarity on your partner.

It's a good idea to have some polarity treatment yourself so that you become aware of the releasing sensations that can occur if you intend to use it on a partner.

THE POLARITY HEAD CRADLE

This is a preparatory treatment to more complex polarities.

1   Have your partner lie flat on his or her back. Place your palms along the sides of their head, the left hand slightly higher.
2   Point your index fingers towards the chest. Your hands should take the shape of the head, softly enclosing but not really holding it.
3   Be relaxed in yourself without trying to feel particularly calm; keep your mind open and associate freely. Don't ask your partner to relax, but occasionally suggest they take a deep breath.
4   Offer your presence to your massage partner, simply being with them, accepting rather than trying to change their condition.
5   Initially, limit a session to five minutes until you get used to this technique. Be sure to take time for your own deep breathing afterwards.

REFLEXOLOGY

Early Egyptian and Chinese civilizations practised reflexology, sometimes called zone therapy. The basis of this technique is that

73

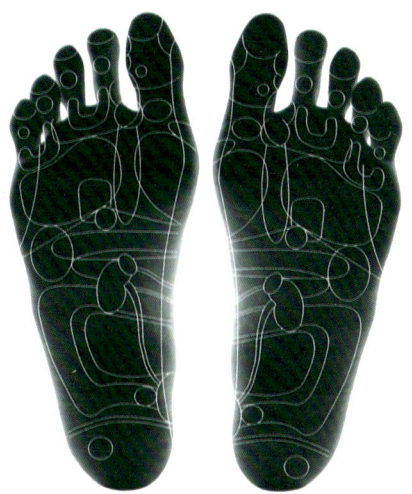

ABOVE IN REFLEXOLOGY, YOUR FEET ARE GIVEN ZONES THAT RELATE TO DIFFERENT AREAS OF THE BODY.

reflex points mapped out on the feet and hands are related to different areas of the body. As we know from everyday experience, the soles of the feet and palms are richly supplied with nerve endings but these are not the same as the reflexes.

The technique is thought to be derived from Chinese acupuncture theory, which is very humanistic compared to rational Western medicine and conceives of a body-energy that includes the personality. The reflexes extend from the extremities to the top of the head along meridians or pathways containing physical and emotional elements of health. By applying pressure on the reflex points, the reflexologist releases congestion along the meridians and improves the functioning of the body organs.

REFLEXOLOGY FOR A STRAINED BACK

If your partner's spinal muscles are in spasm or you are unsure about treating a bad back, try this technique:

1   Have your partner stand sideways, then lie down and compare the silhouette of the foot with that of the spine. I have always found that these will correspond. For example, a long arch of the foot will be reflected in the lumbar spine; a strong curve over the base of the big toe is usually seen as a pronounced curve of the thoracic spine.

2   Place a pillow under the knees and the ankles so that the feet extend. Steady the foot by lightly holding the

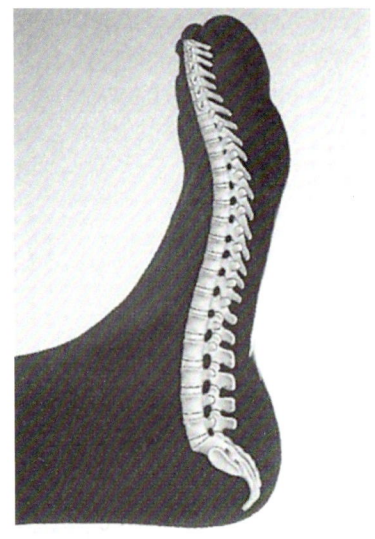

ABOVE THE FOOT IN SILHOUETTE RELATES TO THE SPINAL COLUMN.

toes, and effleurage the instep with the thumb or heel of your hand, with even pressure in both directions.

3   Using the edge of your thumb, trace along the instep and feel for hard points, 'knots' or 'crunches'. These points are usually unexpectedly painful for back sufferers and will reflect as the tightest areas of the spinal column.

4   Using a flatter part of your thumb, keep a steady circling pressure on a painful point as if to rub it away. You will gradually be able to increase pressure, and the pain will lessen. There are normally at least two such strongly sensitive points along the spinal reflex. Spend up to two minutes on each point.

5   Effleurage the instep and treat the other foot.

TIP

You may wash your partner's feet in warm water before the treatment, and your hands in cold water afterwards. If during the massage your hands begin to feel uncomfortable, stop and shake them; this will be a refreshing pause and helpful to your partner. Many people fall asleep during reflexology, so be careful to awaken them by softly calling their name, or gently touching their hand.

SHIATSU

Shiatsu is a Japanese word for finger-pressure massage. Practitioners use their thumbs, elbows and heels to disperse tensions throughout the body. Many Japanese use the services of the visiting shiatsu therapist, and it is common for members of the family to practise on each other.

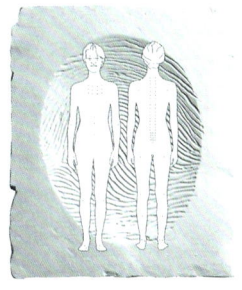

ABOVE IN SHIATSU, PATHWAYS OF ENERGY LINK THE ORGANS.

Shiatsu has a calming influence on hypertensions, and can energize people too low in tension. Many people find it useful for pain relief, and it demonstrates something we already know by instinct – pressure on one tender spot often releases a wider area of tension. The meridians of the Chinese system are thought to operate in shiatsu therapy.

SHIATSU FOR A STIFF SHOULDER

Stand behind your seated partner and ask for some movement in a stiff shoulder. Squeeze gently around the shoulder joint and shoulder bone. It may be that your partner is tender or numb around the shoulder. In regular massage, you would try to loosen up the area with petrissage; instead try the following:

1   Using thumb pressure, move around the whole shoulder, probing deeply. It is very likely that you will discover one or more unexpectedly painful points.
2   Place your thumb (or both thumbs together on a strong shoulder) directly on a point. Ask your partner to breathe out slowly as you press directly into the point for about 10 seconds. Release the pressure gradually as your partner inhales. Explain this beforehand to prepare your partner for such a direct pressure. The formerly painful point will desensitize as they breathe out, and you can encourage them by breathing out in unison. It may also help if they visualize the pain being pressed out of their body.
3   Repeat twice more on other points around the same area.
4   Mobilize the shoulder gently and ask if your partner observes the freer movement.

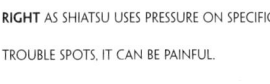

RIGHT AS SHIATSU USES PRESSURE ON SPECIFIC TROUBLE SPOTS, IT CAN BE PAINFUL.

SHIATSU FOR FATIGUE

The shiatsu described here combines with the principles of reflexology for its benefits:

1 Have your partner lie face downwards on a padded floor, a small pillow under their feet, which should be 12 inches apart.
2 Stand, facing away and delicately place your heels on to the soles of their feet.
3 Adding pressure gradually, knead the feet, transferring your weight from foot to foot, for a maximum of 10 minutes.
4 Wrap the feet up to keep them warm, and invite your partner to move into a comfortable position for further relaxation.

TIP

It may be a good idea on the first treatment to wash the feet in warm water first to assist the circulation. This will make the soles supple and might offset the tendency for cramp in the instep due to your pressure being unrelieved. If cramp does occur, stop immediately, extend the big toe and ask your partner to breathe deeply before trying to continue.

RIGHT THIS FORM OF SHIATSU ILLUSTRATES THE HIGH REGARD ORIENTAL CULTURE HAS FOR THE FEET AS HEALING INSTRUMENTS.

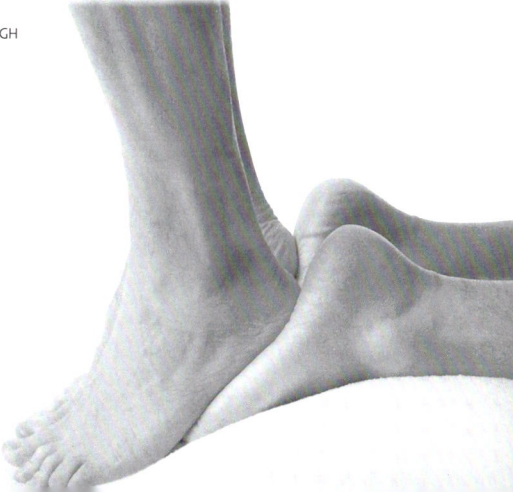

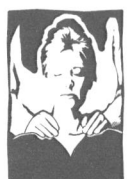

MASSAGE FOR INJURIES

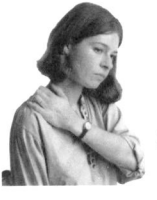

CHAPTER EIGHT

ABOVE WE HAVE A
NATURAL INSTINCT TO
RUB AN INJURED AREA.

Massage has a valuable role to play in helping the body to recover from injury and can be used to complement the body's natural healing process. Knowing when and in what circumstances to use it is vital if it is to be safe and effective.

TYPES OF INJURY

Injuries are a part of everyday life – they record our overexertions. Sometimes we don't notice an injury, like an old bruise that can't be explained. Sometimes an injury takes over our lives; like a bone fracture that can become one of life's major inconveniences. Injuries are traumatic, in that our consciousness registers a reaction to any assault; when we experience this we are said to be 'in shock'. Unlike our illnesses, which often recur, we make complete recoveries from most injuries.

Our reaction to being injured often relates to how much inconvenience it creates. For treatment purposes, injuries can be categorized into two groups: 'trivial', where damage is slight and recovery comes from simple resting; and 'serious', in which there is destruction or discontinuity of tissue, producing disability.

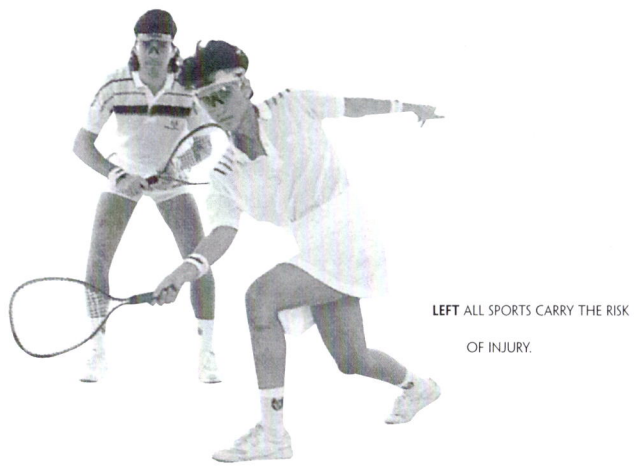

LEFT ALL SPORTS CARRY THE RISK OF INJURY.

TRIVIAL INJURIES

This category often refers to situations as much as to damage, where we assume that our injury is insignificant because of its simple cause. Also, our minor reactions are not always easy to assess; usually there is mild stiffness and some inflammation but if this diminishes after 24 hours, we feel a recovery has been made.

Many trivial injuries are caused by over use of the body, and even if the pressure to use does not relent, interruption and rest usually keep problems at bay. Recurring, seemingly trivial injuries, such as the common bad back, require investigation both of the condition and of the circumstances that provoke it.

SERIOUS INJURIES

An initially trivial injury can develop into a serious injury, but usually it will be apparent from the outset that swelling or loss of blood and pain indicates that some severe damage has occurred. A serious injury does not actually mean it is more life-threatening; in fact, vigorous reaction to injury demonstrates that the body is in full healthy response. More time will be required for healing, and this will give the opportunity to apply the appropriate treatments to optimize the body's effort. This is where massage can be very helpful.

THE BODY'S RESPONSE TO INJURY

Injuries almost inevitably involve loss of blood, since tiny blood vessels are easily ruptured. The escaping blood seeps between layers of body tissue and is further distributed by the effects of gravity. This can explain why a bruise is not always on the painful part. If a significant portion of circulating blood is lost, this can cause a major disturbance in blood pressure, often more serious than the initial injury. Bleeding should always be staunched with cold water, pressure and elevation rather than a tourniquet.

Soon after injury has occurred, the small vessels begin to constrict and the blood clots. This is achieved by the coagulating cells in the blood, the platelets, which help to link body tissue back together again. Unless an injury is aggravated, all this happens quite quickly, so it is wise not to move an injured person unnecessarily, unless they are in a position of greater danger.

REPAIR AND REJUVENATION

An injured person will experience heat, redness, swelling and tenderness in the affected area. This response actually indicates that the healing process is underway. Simultaneous with blood loss is the action of the undamaged structures nearby, which encourage adjacent vessels to dilate and allow blood that is more fluid than usual to arrive at the injury. This blood contains an increased number of white blood cells, leucocytes, which scavenge the injury, and which is termed exudate. The exudate is very effective in disinfecting the injury, helping to stiffen the area and inhibit movement that would complicate the damage. Its presence also stimulates the growth of new tissue.

There is obviously great value in this spontaneous response and because of this, these secondary pains should be borne bravely but massage intervention can alleviate much of the discomfort. Treatment of an injury begins with pain control, and careful management aims to prevent complications.

BELOW UNLESS A PLASTER CAST IS USED, MASSAGE TREATMENT FOR BROKEN BONES

CAN TAKE PLACE DURING AND AFTER THE IMMOBILIZATION OF FRACTURES.

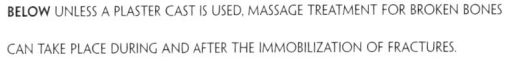

COMMON INJURIES

A seriously injured person should always be taken to the nearest medical services. This is necessary so that all aspects of an injury may be examined properly. The massage treatment described here assumes a competent diagnosis has been

made. If you are ever in the position of handling an injury without medical assistance, you must trust in your own abilities, follow the principles of first aid and proceed with a confidence that will reassure the injured. Here are some common injuries that can be helped by massage.

DISLOCATED JOINTS
A dislocated joint is one that has been forced from its normal position. A relocation is performed by professionals, often under general anaesthetic.

BONE INJURIES
The most serious bone injury is a fracture, ranging from the very simple stress type to very complicated situations where bone fragments interfere with other tissues (such as a rib with a lung). Massage treatments are indicated both during and after the immobilization of fractures.

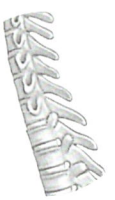

CERVICAL

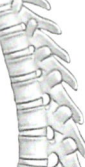

THORACIC

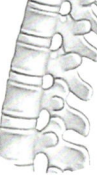

LUMBAR

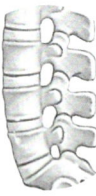

LUMBAR

CARE OF THE SPINE

Fractures of the spine are medical emergencies. Aligned posture rather than exercise is the key to maintaining improvement of spinal problems. It is worth remembering the following tips:

• The spine is central to the body and is designed to make standing up effortless.

• Greater attention to holding on to the muscles of the abdomen is more important than trying to relax a tight back.

• Sitting down produces more strain on the spine than standing upright.

• Gentle walking or lying down with your legs raised and flexed are relaxing positions for the spine.

ABOVE THE CURVE OF THE SPINE ENABLES IT TO ABSORB STRAIN AS YOU WALK AND RUN.

SPINAL INJURIES

These are most likely to take place at recognizable stress points between specialized vertebrae: for instance, from neck to chest, and at the junction of the spine and pelvis. More serious spinal injury involves unacceptable pressure on the discs between the vertebrae, which act as shock absorbers. The discs are designed and accustomed to the varying pressures of posture and are reduced in thickness as the day progresses like cushions on furniture – recovering their shape with rest. With uneven pressure, however, the disc can be squeezed on to adjacent structures such as a spinal nerve, known as a trapped nerve, and the local and radiating pain can be intense.

SPORTS INJURIES

These are experienced because of unfitness, faulty technique and over-enthusiasm. All sports carry a greater risk of injury than everyday life, especially when they are done to offset an unhealthy lifestyle. Sport can make one-sided demands on the body, and stresses in competitive sports sometimes override the benefits of training. Rehabilitation, in the form of special exercises, plays an integral part in massage where the muscles' helpers, the ligaments, which support the joints, have also suffered damage.

83

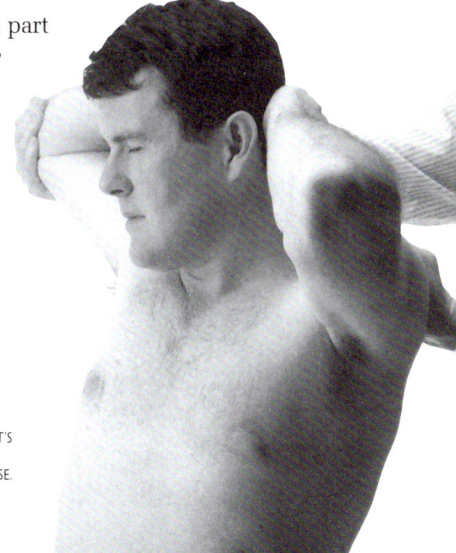

RIGHT OVERUSE OF OUR MUSCLES THROUGH SPORT'S

ACTIVITIES CAN BE AS DAMAGING AS UNDERUSE.

JOINT INJURIES

These usually occur from falls, and range from sprain, where the ligaments are stretched or torn, to dislocation, a serious and violent loss of posture. Often a joint will accept injury to spare the main bone fracturing. This may be expedient in the short term, but joint injuries heal slowly and can have later rheumatic-type difficulties if treated badly, whereas bones almost look after themselves.

Joints are tolerant of slower, extreme pressures while light, jerky movements can easily stretch them. Manipulation techniques make use of this 'quick-snap' principle for therapeutic purposes where joints have become fixated.

Strong, supple muscles are the best protection against joint injuries. Torn ligaments can be repaired surgically, but provided the torn parts are in contact and remain still, healing will occur spontaneously. It has been shown that even a severed Achilles tendon (above the heel) recovers if the parts are simply set against each other.

84

SKIN INJURIES

These include abrasions, lacerations, burns and scalds. All these injuries respond favourably to the application of hydrotherapy (*see* p.67). The skin has three layers: the epidermis, dermis and subcutis. It is an extremely regenerative organ and you will have noticed that superficial scratches to the epidermis often recover completely within 48 hours.

For deeper wounds, hydrotherapy treatment provides the ideal conditions for effective pain relief, as well as cleansing and protecting the wound. Burns that penetrate the skin or cover a major portion of its surface require complex medical attention because of the skin's important organic functions, but even then the application of moisture is regarded as a helpful aid to recovery. Another benefit from using hydrotherapy for skin wounds is that stitching may be avoided, and deeper cleansing is possible, which discourages scarring.

MUSCLE AND TENDON INJURIES

These include tears, ruptures and strains. Muscles protect as well as move the body, and are called upon to make heroic rescues. Muscle tissue receives extraordinary energy at times of danger, but our underlying level of fitness will determine our body's speed of reaction. Certain sports and occupations, however, call for development of one set of muscles beyond others, and many injuries result from this imbalance.

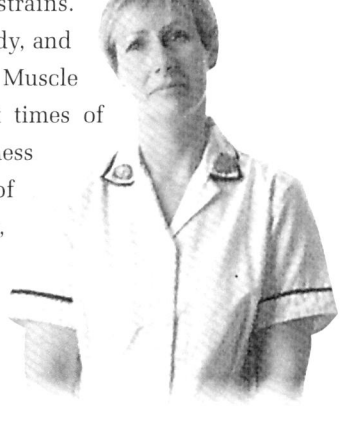

Serious muscle injury requires complete rest of that muscle, and if we find it hard to resist moving, we can end up in a plaster cast. Though effective as a prison and punishment, this is not

ABOVE PHYSIOTHERAPY IS AN IMPORTANT PART OF TREATING MUSCLE INJURIES.

85

necessarily helpful to the injury, which tends to get isolated from the body to which it rightfully belongs. Recurring injuries in fit people suggest an inappropriate choice of sport, and within teams people have to be careful to play in positions that suit their physique. With increased leisure facilities and emphasis on sport and health, increased demand for injury treatment from health professionals such as physiotherapists is predicted.

TREATING INJURIES

The management of an injury consists of three stages. These stages of treatment are:
- Limitation of its disturbance (2–8 hours).
- Encouraging circulation; massage (after 24–48 hours).
- Rehabilitation exercise (until normality restored).

We will now look at the example of how an injured ankle would be treated.

STAGE 1: LIMITATION OF THE INJURY

This is achieved with compression bandages and cold water. The body's immediate reaction to injury is to produce exudate, the specialized blood that stimulates healing and cleanses the wound. It is important to restrict the amount of exudate by containing the injury from without; this discourages too much exudate forming and prevents stickiness around the injury which could give rise to adhesions. Adhering tissues create stiffness after healing and cause pain. They cannot be broken down later by massage and, if serious, will require surgery.

Another possible cause of adhesion is massage or exercise too early in the repair of an injury. Premature movement irritates damaged tissue and causes more exudate to form.

APPLYING A COMPRESSION BANDAGE

As soon as possible after the injury, surround the ankle with layers of cotton wool and a crepe bandage, with the wool interspersed between the turns of the bandage.

The injury should then be immersed or soaked in ice-cold water for 15 minutes. Cold helps relieve pain by reducing the conductivity of the nerves, and constricts the capillaries of the superficial structures to prevent further blood loss. For these reasons, never apply heat to an injury in the acute stage. Hot application is best used later to relieve muscle spasm and increase the blood supply to the injury.

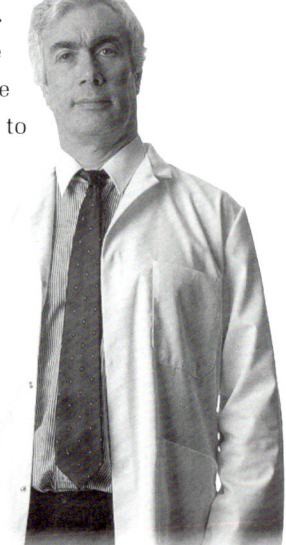

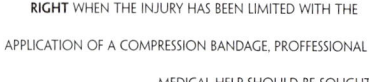
RIGHT WHEN THE INJURY HAS BEEN LIMITED WITH THE APPLICATION OF A COMPRESSION BANDAGE, PROFFESSIONAL MEDICAL HELP SHOULD BE SOUGHT.

The bandage is intended to hold the area in a firm support but with the structure in a neutral, anatomical posture. Slightly flex knees and elbows but fully flex ankle injuries towards the knee. If possible, place the injury higher than chest level. The bandage should be kept wet and cold. At this point consideration can be given as to how to deliver the injured person to the medical services. Once diagnosis has been obtained, or if no services are available, continue with stage 2.

STAGE 2: ENCOURAGING THE CIRCULATION

Within 36–48 hours, most soft tissue injuries have established healing reactions. The aim of treatment now is to encourage the circulation around the injury and to keep the body comfortably at rest. Remove the bandage and inspect the ankle. (If there is no significant reduction of swelling, the bandage is replaced wet and cold for a further 24 hours.)

If the swelling has reduced but the injury is still painful use self-massage or contrast hydrotherapy.

87

SELF-MASSAGE

Ask your partner to make active movements above and below the injury; in the case of the ankle, knee flexing and toe wriggling for two minutes. Avoid direct irritation and preferably have the leg raised. An infra-red (radiant) heat lamp can sometimes be used at this stage.

CONTRAST HYDROTHERAPY

Apply a very hot towel and then a cold one for three minutes each, six times, ending with cold. A spray of hot and cold water can be used instead.

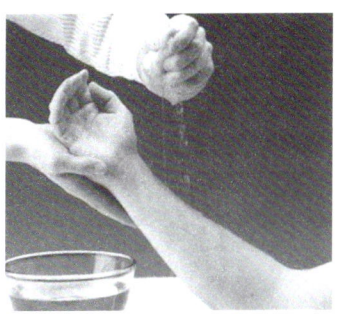

Note: If the injury includes a burn or cut, omit the hot application and alternate cold with three minutes rest.

ABOVE COOL WATER HYDROTHERAPY IS IDEAL FOR CERTAIN INJURIES, SUCH AS FRACTURES.

Replace the compression bandage. A wet bandage should not be kept on overnight but the injury can be dry bandaged and kept cool by a surrounding wet towel. If painful during the night, the ankle should be cold plunged but not dried before re-applying the bandage. The night bandage should be soaked off in the morning.

MASSAGE

If, after 48 hours, the injury has improved to the extent that swelling and tenderness is reduced, you may then begin gentle hand massage. If not, repeat the stages above.

Swelling that has not diminished indicates deeper damage, possibly to a bone or, not uncommonly, overuse by the injured. If your partner has experienced emotional shock as well as injury, these early stages can take longer to pass.

1   Repeat the hot and cold applications. Make strong effleurage up to (not over) the injury, then continue beyond. Repeat until there is further visible reduction in swelling.

2   Ask for some tentative movements around the injury for two minutes. Support the area with dry cotton wool and a crepe bandage and suggest your partner make normal use of their body, with rest periods throughout the day. The injury can be cold plunged when painful.

3   Two days later, if the swelling is further diminished: effleurage up to, then lightly over the ankle and firmly beyond. Friction stroke over the injury; circling with your finger tips, aiming to gently loosen rather than penetrate the skin. You may lightly oil your fingers with lavender blended essential oil, if your partner agrees. Repeat effleurage.

These strokes discourage the formation of adhesions from the circulatory response to the injury. They are not intended to disturb the healing process that is taking place in the new tissues. To assist in circulatory return, have the injury elevated or packed up on pillows during and after the massage.

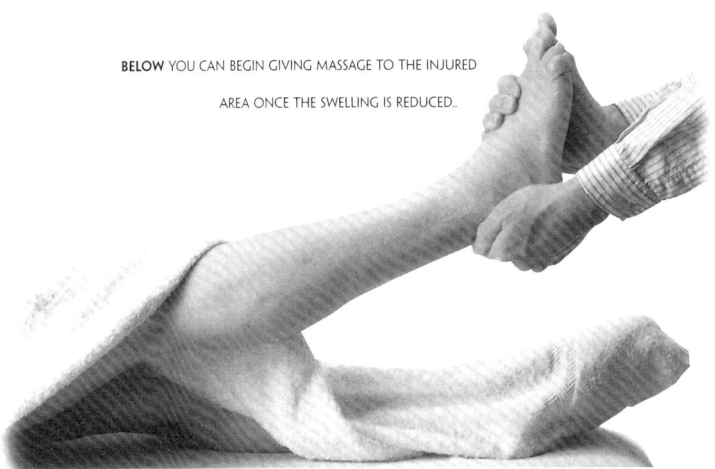

BELOW YOU CAN BEGIN GIVING MASSAGE TO THE INJURED AREA ONCE THE SWELLING IS REDUCED..

Depending on the severity of the injury, massages can be continued every other day until your partner regains confidence in using the injured part. The dry bandage can be worn until the swelling disappears completely but should be removed overnight.

STAGE 3: REHABILITATION

When near normal use of the injured part is achieved, an exercise programme is introduced after massage. (General body massage may be given after the first 24 hours of the injury. Apart from the relaxation benefits, particular attention can be given to areas that are compensating for the inconvenience of the injury – opposite leg, shoulders, and so on.)

The exercises have three aims: to improve strength, flexibility and co-ordination. They also have three styles: passive, active and resistive.

BUILDING STRENGTH

Perform these exercises on alternate days.

- Passive exercise: hold the foot carefully and move it around, reminding your partner of their ankle's movements.
- Active exercise: ask your partner to move the ankle slowly and deliberately.

- Resistive: hold the foot firmly. Ask your partner to move the ankle as before, trying (but not desperately) to overcome your resistance. Aim to balance out each other's tension. Rest and repeat until fatigued (not the massager!)

INCREASING FLEXIBILITY

Injured tissues contract and lose tone while repairing. Stretches are introduced to regain elasticity and further improve circulation. Increased flexibility is not easy to measure unless you have known your partner's condition before injury. Comparison with non-injured sides of the body may guide you.

- Passive: demonstrate stretching by pointing, flexing and twisting the foot, holding at extreme position for three seconds.
- Active: ask your partner to repeat the movements slowly.
- Resistive: ask your partner to point the foot against your resistance; both agree to relax and immediately move the joint smoothly in the opposite direction to its comfortable limit.
- Repeat flexing and twisting to both sides.

IMPROVING CO-ORDINATION

Exercises in co-ordination help to reintegrate an injury with the rest of the body. This involves a kind of reclaiming of a limb or posture by your partner, and it can often be an emotional experience. When treating a partner always be aware that your role is to encourage rather than coerce, and as you perform the massage, give constant reassurance.

- Passive: walk backwards, sideways etc. Demonstrate the movement you are proposing. Go slowly and repeat if necessary.
- Active: have your partner pass something (for instance, a ball), from foot to foot; play music and move in rhythm.
- Resistive: ask your partner to stop in mid-step; change direction quickly as requested; balance on one leg, and so on.

STAYING POSITIVE AND PATIENT

Creativity with the exercise programme provides interest and stimulation for your partner's energy to recover. Injuries can involve emotional depression and oscillation between over-enthusiasm and despair. Your consistency in positively anticipating a satisfactory and realistic outcome to the injury is also vital.

Most injuries to the soft tissues (that is, the skin, muscles and ligaments of the joints of the limbs) can be treated along the lines of the above example. Trunk injuries are more complicated to manage due to greater nervous involvement. Injuries, like their owners, can be unpredictable, and you will develop

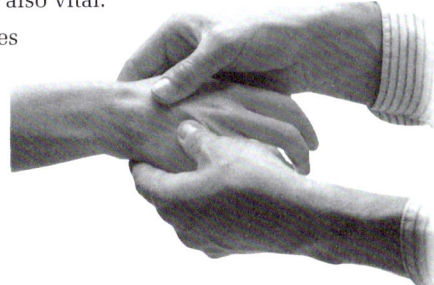

ABOVE A POSITIVE AND CREATIVE APPROACH TO YOUR PARTNER'S TREATMENT WILL SPEED RECOVERY.

91

tremendous patience as well as admiration while attending to your partner's healing processes. If you are in doubt about any aspect of a recovery, consult an experienced practitioner.

PREDISPOSITION TO INJURY

Our injuries possibly teach us more about ourselves than our illnesses do. The fact that recoveries are usually so complete distinguishes injuries from most disease processes. Having experienced injury, we learn how to avoid problems, whereas illness and the reasons we are given for its cause have relatively little effect on its incidence, if the major diseases of today are considered. (Ironically, the more we appreciate about modern diseases, such as heart disease, the more they begin to sound like self-inflicted injuries.)

Factors that are associated with injury include our level of fitness, how tired we are, our diet and what we prefer to call 'accidents'.

FITNESS

It is hard to find a definition of fitness with which everyone agrees. The condition of our lungs and heart are partly inherited; there are those who are advantaged by a better start in life, while others falter in spite of their healthy resolutions.

Although we are beginning to recognize activities that are potentially damaging, some people, not unreasonably, wonder just what we are preserving ourselves for, if not to enjoy a measure of indulgence! The attitude 'as fit as I need to be' may be more philosophical than complacent, and reflects the attitude of someone curled up, relaxed with a book and a cigarette, compared with a panting, defeated executive on an electronic cycling machine. A truly unfit person confidently knows what their limitations are.

TIREDNESS AND TENSION

These can be two sides of the same coin, which suggests strain and pushing up to and beyond tolerable limits. Sometimes it would appear that tiredness is offered as a sign of commitment to our work or family, yet there is no doubt that our reflexes and reactions are dulled by excessive tension.

Those who go unscathed from going 'all out' may succeed by making distinct changes in direction – work hard/play hard collapse/bounce back again. Effective, perhaps, but in ways other people find too demanding as a route to relaxation.

DIET

Malnourishment means poor growth and consequently poor repair. Affluent societies suffer not only from refined, impoverished food but from the complexity of a rich diet that takes as much energy to consume as it gives, and over-consumption of even wholesome food can still result in a net loss in nutrition.

Perhaps the most researched and demonstrable dietary factor associated with injury is the way some foods undermine body efficiency. Processed foods slow up healing, while fasting accelerates it; stimulating foods deplete energy; popular weight-reducing diets contradict natural appetite.

Among the many controversies surrounding diet, confusion over fluid intake persists. Earlier recommendations to drink at least four litres per day have given way by 50 per cent but this is still at variance with present physiological knowledge; beyond a small amount, water requirements, like food, are relative to the individual's make up. There is evidence to show that a high intake of any fluid disturbs digestion and depletes strength. The high salt content of the processed foods we eat also results in a tendency to retain fluid in the body. Body builders are careful to drink very little for days before a contest, which may suggest that a moderate consumption of fluids is the healthy course.

93

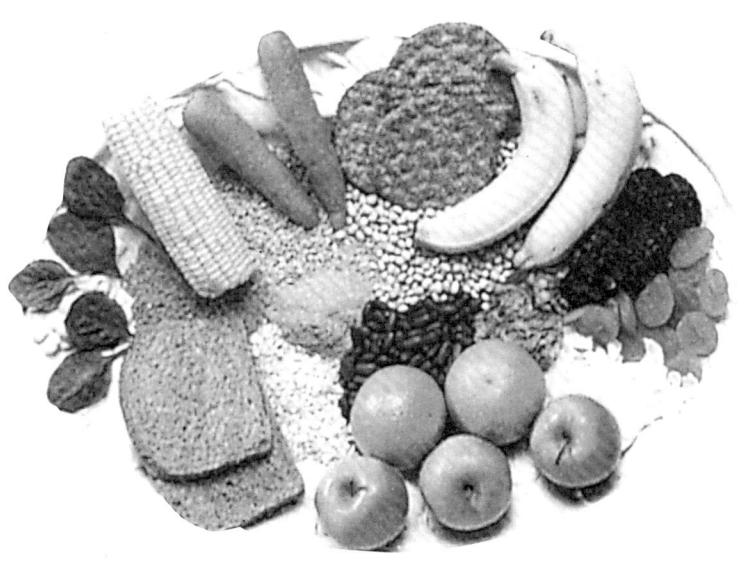

ABOVE EATING FRESH RATHER THAN PROCESSED FOODS

PROVIDES YOU WITH THE MOST NUTRITIOUS DIET.

'ACCIDENTS'

How would you define an accident? Are you able to find a definition that still makes you feel secure in the world? Perfectly trained, perfectly relaxed and perfectly nourished people incur injury, and when it happens we routinely call this an accident. There is an assumption that accidents are unexpected, unavoidable and somehow unfair. For the majority of us this prospect does not prevent our wholehearted involvement in many intense, high-risk activities. We are increasingly aware of the emotional investments in many illnesses. Do they also apply in the case of injuries? Perhaps not in the sense that being shipwrecked or present at an earthquake suggests the unavoidable nature of certain accidents. We do however hear accounts of the uncanny coincidences associated with such events.

'Accident prone', an expression hinting that we might have a tendency to fall into injury in relatively innocent circumstances, is a condition many will have experienced at some time in life. What gets injured at these times can be as intriguing as why it should have happened.

94

A NEW APPROACH TO INJURY

One positive way of facing the likelihood of injury might be to have regular modifications of the treatment that we know produces reliable healing as a preventative. This follows a traditional edict in natural therapy: 'The care is the cure and the cure is the care.'

This approach allows you to offer as part of your massages, emphasis on the containing, mobilizing and supportive elements of injury treatment. The methods are best learned on uninjured partners so as to have developed confidence for injuries when they arise.

CONTAINMENT

The enforced rest of the massage session is the element equivalent to the use of a compression bandage: the body is immobilized, heat distributed and gravity offset. Many partners will become accustomed to the regularity of treatment but for someone who finds it easier to 'keep going than to stop', an enforced rest is unappealing; your massage strokes will have to justify your persuasion.

Less active partners will look forward to their treatment as a relief, and make their appointments well in to the future. While the former may follow your suggestion and take a holiday but be un-communicative, the latter would send a postcard: a massage message. For everyone, massage offers an interruption of what we become habituated to and helps us avoid some of the damage that otherwise it would be impossible to avoid.

EMOTIONAL SUPPORT THROUGH MASSAGE

Quite often emotional trauma can precede physical injury and, although I have described some injuries as 'trivial', we should take care not to minimize someone's feelings. Life's events affect people in unique ways and sometimes result in conflicting responses. Expressions of conflict such as grief and resentment are legitimate within treatment, leaving partners freer to respond, if, as practitioners, we are able to accept them.

The challenge is not to pacify immediately but to let our partner interpret the strokes in a supportive atmosphere. Regular massages punctuate the hidden strains of life, and the knowledge that someone is maintaining an informed interest in our condition continues that support.

ABOVE NEGATIVE EMOTIONS CAN EMERGE DURING TREATMENT.

MOBILIZING

Our partners may not always appreciate our interest in the extremely tense areas of their body, since attention to a problem is not always as pleasant as a general treatment. However, as observers of what partners may be only vaguely aware of, we are obliged to attempt to free tension and unblock the circulation of the body. Always be as supportive as possible. Great care is required to investigate deep tensions, as we have to avoid giving our partners the impression that they are in a worse state than they thought!

Your affinity with your partner's structure, and the personal rapport between you should allow you to introduce treatments that you consider would be helpful. (This is how practices mature, as partners come to rely on your feelings about their body as much as they do their own.)

Given the unexpectedness of injury, the mobilization movements of massage can become a part of your general treatments. Familiarization with the anatomy of joints will enable you to exercise the structures that strengthen them. Experiment and create your own rehabilitation programme. Very tired partners will be surprised to discover how stimulating the exercises can be.

LEFT PERSONAL RAPPORT BETWEEN THE PERSON "GIVING" AND THE PERSON "RECEIVING" IS IMPORTANT.

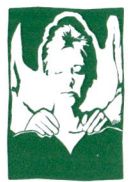

SELF-MASSAGE AS FIRST AID

There may be occasions when treatment for an injury is needed before you have the opportunity to get help from a friend or practitioner – emergencies rarely occur in ideal treatment conditions. When your immediate need is to cope well with your situation until expert help is available, I recommend the following self-help tips. These procedures have been tried and tested in a variety of circumstances – on a desert island, in homes and in high-tech hospital wards. You never know when you may find them useful.

PREVENTATIVE ACTION

While the information I give in this chapter is primarily intended as first aid, you can use these 'coping strategies' equally effectively as preventative actions. By including them as part of your health maintenance regime, it might be possible to avoid the build-up conditions that often precede an emergency such as a disabling muscle spasm experienced in the back.

When you have experienced first aids on yourself, I am sure that you will be confident to offer many of them to a friend in need – hopefully, not all in the same day!

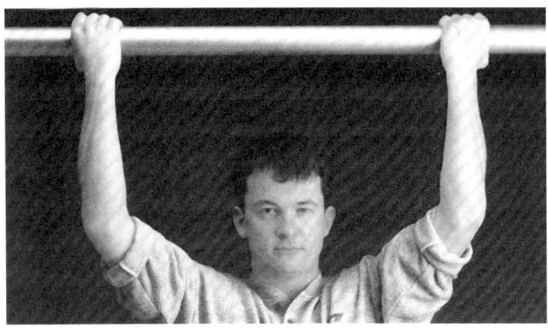

LEFT THE WHOLE BODY STRETCH IS ESPECIALLY BENEFICIAL IN THE EARLY AFTERNOON WHEN THE BODY IS BEGINNING TO TIRE.

RELAXATION FOR THE WHOLE BODY

A very obvious, though not widely adopted, way to minimize everyday strain is demonstrated by our domestic animals:

- Simple when it's not essential to stand up – sit down, with the knees well flexed; if sitting is uncomfortable – lie down, with the spine curled.

Some might feel that circumstances and convention constrain their attempts to follow this first aid. However, alternatives such as standing with the weight on one leg, sagging or crossing one leg over the other from a chair are all token indications that the body is weary and is probably reflecting our feelings about the situation in which we find ourselves. It might improve a situation more than interrupt it if a brief resting posture can be found. Here is a useful, fleeting alternative to recumbence.

1   Find a doorway with a surround deep enough to allow you to reach up and hold on. (In modern houses and offices it might be insufficient; sports' shops sell a telescopic hand-hold which can be adjusted to fit a door space and you might be advised to invest in one as a consideration for both your body and the door.)

2   Hold tight but relax your arms straight. Let your arms bend slowly as you take up your weight through the arms.

3   Breathing out, imagine that you are sitting down on to a stool you can't quite reach. You'll feel the muscles of the trunk lengthening.

Let your knees bend naturally and keep your feet in contact with the floor.

4   As you feel your whole body stretching out, you can swing your knees gently from side to side, head slightly dropping forward.

5   When your grip begins to tire, draw your abdomen in firmly and put your weight back on to your feet and stand up slowly.

You can do this whenever you sense tension or tiredness in your body or in a situation, but later in the afternoon is the optimum time for many people.

SELF-MASSAGE FOR THE BACK

For no immediately apparent reasons, backs sometimes 'go'. There is usually a split-second awareness of something not quite right in our posture, followed by a seizing of all the muscles in the vicinity, if not the whole body.

Although essentially defensive in its reaction, the dramatic rise in muscular tension is very unnerving. Sometimes the body seems to freeze and be incapable of any more movement at all without assistance, but for most people there is an overwhelming urge to relieve the weight from the spine.

Back emergencies are such universal experiences that many intuitive and original first aids have been developed. The following is suggested for any situation involving seizure of the lower and upper back muscles.

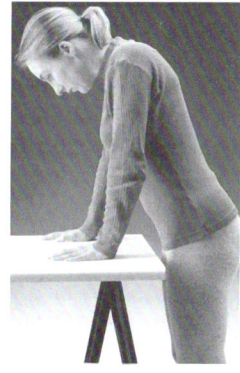

1   As soon as a problem arises (for instance, from lifting, twisting, falling, and so on), place the body weight forwards, on to the hands; lean on to furniture, or if severe, get down on all fours.

ABOVE AS SOON AS YOU EXPERIENCE A BACK PROBLEM, PLACE YOUR WEIGHT ON YOUR HANDS.

2 Breathe deeply (oxygen helps relieve spasm) and try to assess the sensation. It is very likely that one side of the back is primarily affected and is involving other nearby muscles. Ask someone to look at your posture, which will show obvious deviation to the primary tension. If alone, move gently to the left or right.

3 When you have decided which side is affected (no need to worry about being absolutely right at this point), lie down on the edge of the body on that side and by degrees draw the opposite knee, up as high as possible to rest your weight upon. Let your elbow on the same side take the upper body weight and turn your head in that direction.

4 Keep the other arm on the opposite side of your body. This should allow you to breathe deeply again and you can check if your back feels easier. (If you have mistaken the side of greater tension, the above will be extremely uncomfortable, though not damaging, and you can slowly and reliably turn over to the correct side.)

5 Rest for a few minutes, reassuring your back muscles by carrying out regular, deep, controlled contractions of your abdomen and by imagining the whole of your trunk being compressed towards the earth by the force of gravity.

6 If feeling easier, very carefully return to the all-fours position. Try to straighten your spine to an upright position by climbing up a piece of furniture, but stay on your knees. If another spasm occurs, return to the former position for a few more minutes.

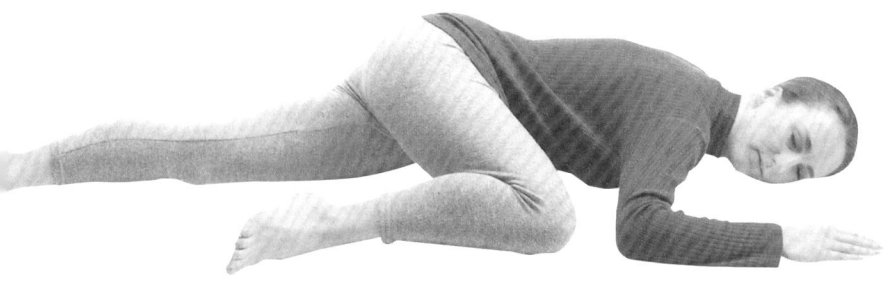

ABOVE YOU'LL FIND THAT THE RECOVERY POSITION HELPS TO RELEASE YOUR BACK MUSCLES.

7   Trying again, make your way to seek assistance, preferably on
    your hands and knees, and then wait for help in the former
    horizontal position.

Don't feel defeated if this procedure is not immediately successful;
you will probably have reduced your pain and certainly have
minimized the work your practitioner will need to do with you. You
may recognize the horizontal position as very similar to the
"recovery" position of conventional first aid, and expectant mothers
may remember it as a relief from pressure on the growing abdomen.

SELF-MASSAGE FOR THE NECK

Problems with our neck muscles can be very psychological but the
neck, although exquisitely designed, is a vulnerable structure: heels
on our shoes cause the head to tilt backwards and shorten the neck;
most of us hear better from one ear and consequently twist the neck
around to the clearer side; violent movements such as car collisions,
while sparing the vertebrae, may tear at the neck's delicate nerves and
blood vessels. This in turn may lead to referred pains in the arms.

The joints of the neck are normally very flexible but when
continually misaligned, compensatory tensions build up around the
bones (often heard as 'crackling' during neck exercises). The neck
may eventually have to be manipulated and exercises followed to
restore posture.

If you would like to encourage a relaxed centredness of your neck
try this:

1   Roll up a small towel to make a diameter of approximately
    three inches.
2   Lie flat on your back with your feet drawn up to stand near
    the buttocks.
3   Place the towel under your neck, not your head, so that the
    normal inward curvature of your neck fits neatly over the towel.
    Relax your jaw.

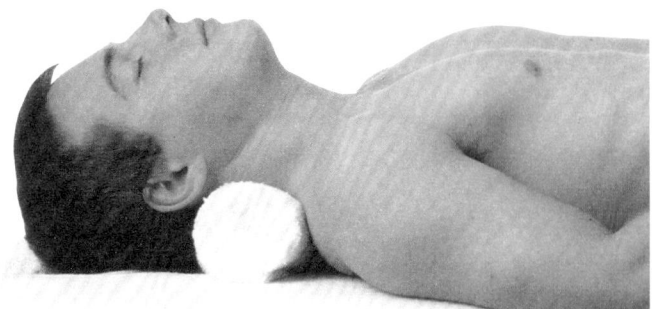

4. Roll the head slightly from side to side against the towel. If one side of the neck feels tighter, roll the head into the stiffness for a few seconds, then slowly roll as far as possible in the opposite direction. Rest. Your neck should feel supported while the tight muscles stretch lightly. Breathe deeply and relax the jaw again.

5. Roll the head slowly back to the centre and relax completely. Lie on one side and push with your arms to become upright. Move your head around lightly.

Discomfort in the face and eyes benefit from this treatment. For sinus-type congestion, apply a hot cloth over the cheeks, and a cold cloth to the feet during the procedure.

SELF-MASSAGE FOR THE ABDOMEN

Pains in the abdomen can mean something very serious since our organs are normally relatively insensitive (Gandhi, the founder of modern India, is reputed to have had his appendix removed without anaesthetic). Before we can assume anything dire, however, we should consider that acute abdominal discomfort is usually the result of indigestion.

Two common causes are eating foods together that can be incompatible, such as fats and starches, and eating when anxious, thereby lacking the necessary digestive juices.

102

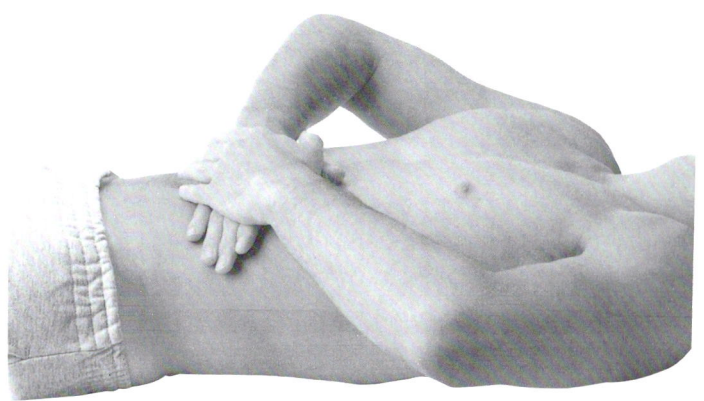

ABOVE WHEN YOU BEGIN MASSAGING THE ABDOMEN INVESTIGATE THE PROBLEM AREA GENTLY.

The pressure that builds up in the intestines from these conditions may be substantial but can be relieved. I was able to congratulate someone on the spontaneous discovery of this first aid. He was a driven, anxious person who ate like a carnivore, and usually on the run: 'I regularly got a pain in my abdomen and I always felt I should press on it. One day I did and it went away. It doesn't happen so often now but the pressing still works.'

1. Lie down with knees bent up. The area around your pain may feel hard. Rub gently with the heel of your hand.
2. Increase the pressure until you feel your abdomen softening. Find the painful spot with your fingertips and slowly begin to press through as if towards the spine.
3. You may detect a release or gurgle and increased relaxation of the abdomen. Rub again in a clockwise direction.
4. Draw your knees up towards your chest and hold on with your hands. Relax and breathe deeply.

Reflux (acid) from the stomach back to the mouth might suggest the beginning of conditions in the upper digestive system that you should consult your practitioner about.

103

SELF-MASSAGE FOR CONSTIPATION

When we are upset, our nervous system is affected and our intestines function erratically, leading to constipation. A simple self-massage technique can help.

1   Practise squatting by holding on to a friend or door handle and lowering your hips between your feet. Try to keep the feet flat.

2   Relax your neck forwards and practise retracting your abdomen, holding back for a few seconds at a time.

3   When you have made your hips more supple, proceed to the toilet seat. Squat on the unit as you have been practising. If you can't manage this without fear of falling, sit down and raise your feet on a box so that your knees are higher than your hips.

4   Retract and slowly release your abdomen a few times.

5   Make a fist and massage deeply around your abdomen, especially on the left side.

6   Relax and breathe deeply. Avoid bearing down, and don't try to empty the bowel which should be an unconscious action. After a few minutes, success or not, get up. Repeat the procedure throughout the day if necessary.

Consult a practitioner if you suffer from abdominal problems that do not respond to first aids.

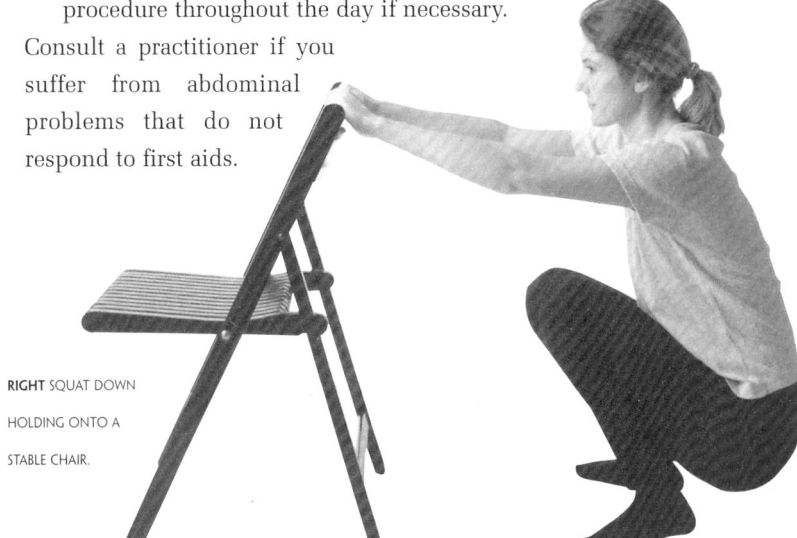

RIGHT SQUAT DOWN
HOLDING ONTO A
STABLE CHAIR.

SELF-MASSAGE FOR MENSTRUAL PAINS

Contrary to some views that would have women do no physical activity at this time. menstrual discomfort can be relieved by simply inverting the pelvis. This position lessens gravity's magnification of symptoms and is pleasantly relaxing for the abdomen and legs, which also become pressurized. If practiced throughout the cycle it may bring a long-term improvement.

1   Lie down with your knees slightly bent. Roll up on to your shoulders and using your elbows as props, support your hips with open hands.
2   When steady, move your legs around slowly and rotate your ankles and flex your toes.
3   Breathe slowly and observe your abdomen go in and out as you breathe.
4   Remain in the position as long as comfortable, for a maximum of one minute. Recover very gradually, avoiding bumping on your spine and pelvis, by bracing your hands against the floor as you roll down.
5   When your spine is flat on the ground, hug your knees to your chest for 10 seconds.
6   Don't get up straight away; you could follow this with light abdominal massage.

105

I include this first aid on the recommendation of female colleagues. It can be done before, during and after the period; consider this an important time to take care of your posture. If you are unsure about how to invert your body, consult a Yoga teacher.

RIGHT WITH PRACTICE YOU CAN ACHIEVE A MORE
UPRIGHT POSITION.

SELF-MASSAGE FOR TIRED EYES

In everyday life our eyes tend to dominate our other senses; we even use the expression 'I see' when understanding something not necessarily connected with looking.

Increased pressures on the eyes cause them to sting, blur and ache; internally the eyes are very responsive to changes in nervous energy and the emotions. In spite of this, their powers of recovery are acute and they do not appear to suffer from overuse (except in monotonous gaze and focusing).

This first aid, called 'palming', rests the eyes and relaxes the neck muscles that are concerned with their effective circulation.

1   Sit close to a table and loosen the clothes from around your neck.
2   Place your palms (not fingers) over the eyes so that no light can enter. Lean forward and rest your elbows on the table.
3   Your hands should almost completely support your head. (Notice how tense the neck muscles become when you lift your head back slightly.) Let your face sink into your hands.
4   Have a mental picture of a vivid, colourful scene, with changing perspectives; 'look' with your physical eyes, exercising your eyes as if the image was outside your body.

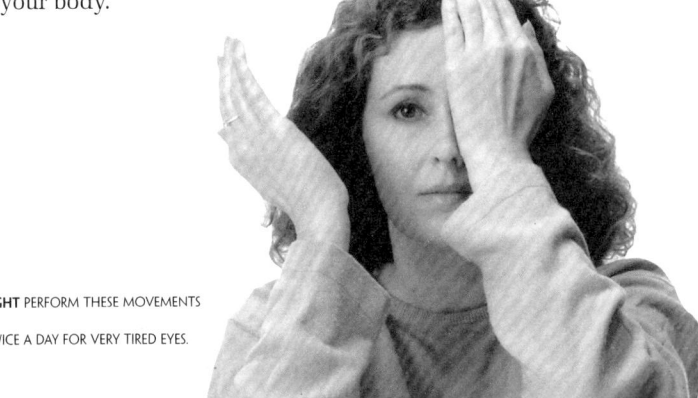

RIGHT PERFORM THESE MOVEMENTS TWICE A DAY FOR VERY TIRED EYES.

5   After a minute, let the image fade, and relax your eyes into the darkness of your palms. Breathe deeply six times.

6   With eyes closed, slowly sit up straight and 'wash' your face with your hands, drawing away from the centre to the sides of the face. Open your eyes gradually.

If you are concerned about your eyes for any reason, do this twice a day and have neck massage.

SELF-MASSAGE FOR THE FEET

Our feet are confined almost from birth in a way that no other part of our body would accept. This is not always for protection and, by the time we realize this, irreversible compensations may have taken place – fallen arches and toe deviations to name the most common. It seems a pity to deny the feet their place in an otherwise relaxed body, and free-moving feet are themselves a great assistance to other disorders, for example, by providing significant help in preventing heart disease and assisting post-operative circulation.

107

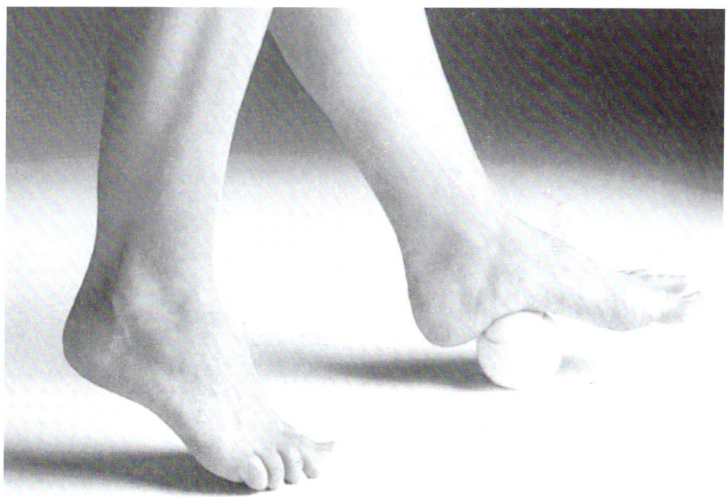

ABOVE FALLEN ARCHES ARE A COMMON RESULT OF ILL-FITTING SHOES.

Choose from this selection of 'feet firsts' or do them all.

1   Take off your shoes and socks. Creep the feet forwards and backwards using clawing actions of the toes; rise up on tiptoe; curl the toes back as far as possible and hold till aching.

2   Put a rubber ball under the foot and roll it backwards and forwards along the instep. Run ankle-deep water in the bath and paddle for three minutes.

3   Play a cold shower as strongly as you can bear on the soles of each foot and against the calves for two minutes. Don't dry the feet but wrap them in a towel and lie down with your legs raised.

These aids also sometimes help with headaches. The water sessions are also useful when you are feeling low or just getting back on your feet after illness.

SELF-MASSAGE FOR INSOMNIA

Sleeplessness, while disturbing, is not regarded as fatal and if we can't get off to sleep or stay asleep we need to develop the same philosophical view as the constipated. Sleeping is not something we do but rather comes over us; often the real complaint is being awake to ourselves, our thoughts and sensations best forgotten for a time. There is also the irony that for some who do eventually get off to sleep, they are unable to wake clearly in the morning.

SELF-HELP FOR EMOTIONAL SHOCK

1   Find a soft place, lie down, and slightly curl up. Hold yourself by folding your arms around the chest and abdomen. Do not squeeze as you need to be able to breathe easily.

2   Occasionally relax your arms and move your toes and fingers for a few seconds. Repeat until you feel more comfortable.

This aid is another form of hydrotherapy.

1   Be ready for bed and go to the wash basin.
2   Run cold tap water over your hands and forearms until they are chilled but not numb.
3   Do not dry your arms but mop your skin and go to bed.
4   Adopt your chosen sleeping position and put your hands between your arms and chest.
5   Forget your desire to sleep, and lie still, breathing deeply. Goodnight.

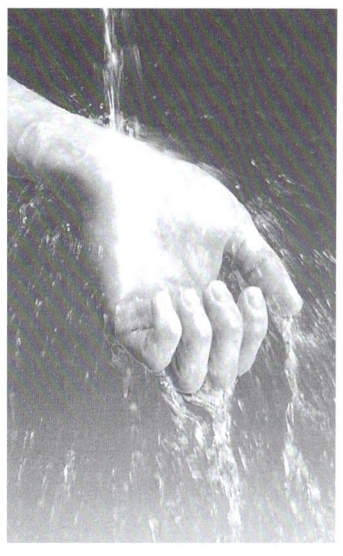

ABOVE WET YOUR HANDS WITH COLD WATER.

109

SELF-HELP FOR PHYSICAL SHOCK

1   Assuming there is no bleeding, seize the injured part in both hands, if available, and compress it as firmly as possible for three minutes. If there is bleeding, apply a pad first, and if glass is in the cut, compress around it.

2   Bind with a cold cloth and avoid weight bearing. If the pain lasts more than 12 hours seek advice.

This is an obvious treatment for a sprain, minimizing swelling and pain. Avoid moving the area until comfortable, otherwise a more serious condition could develop. Massage above and below, and breathe deeply.

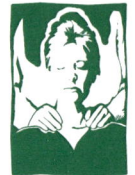

TAKING MASSAGE FURTHER

CHAPTER TEN

Of all the therapies introduced to me as a student naturopathic practitioner, I found that therapeutic touching was the most revolutionary. Up until that time, I had only experienced the cool detachment of the family doctor, and I associated the physiotherapies with infirmity. I subsequently learned that this had not always been so in healthcare, and today among my favourite written resources are massage textbooks that were published at the turn of the century.

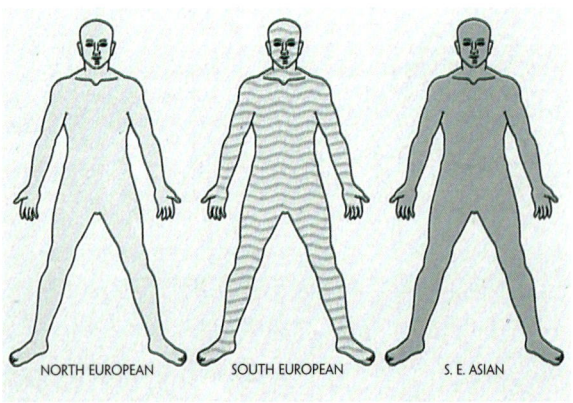

NORTH EUROPEAN   SOUTH EUROPEAN   S. E. ASIAN

ABOVE MASSAGE IS MORE COMMONLY PRACTISED IN PLACES WHERE BODY CONTACT IS PART OF THE CULTURE. THE
DEGREE OF SHADING ON THESE FIGURES INDICATES THE FREQUENCY OF PHYSICAL CONTACT IN THE CULTURE.

During my studies in Edinburgh I came across an article in the London *Sunday Times* from the 1970s that reported on the extent of physical contact between adults throughout the world. Figure diagrams, shaded red for contact, blue for little or none, showed that the further from the equator the less contact occurred. In Scotland, the blue was only relieved by a token smattering of red on hands, head and genitals!

I tried to reconcile these findings with the positive response of patients to massage at the clinic. Everyone seemed to look forward to their treatment and regretted that this would be what they missed most on their return home. For many reasons but perhaps most importantly, accessibility, therapeutic massage was hard to find. Formerly, professional practitioners were indeed few and far between; today the practice of massage is enjoying a well-deserved revival among everyone who is enthusiastic to live a healthy life.

However, because of the associations between massage and prostitution, because massage continues to be confused with physiotherapy and because it is almost easier to admit to having migraine than a massage in our culture, there are still some problems to be overcome. I will discuss some of the issues that come up for people attending introductory massage courses with their friends and family, and describe professional training opportunities for those wishing to make a serious study of massage.

KEEP PRACTISING

For many enthusiasts, lack of practice hinders the development of their massage. Curiously, for new massagers, friends seem to prefer paying a stranger for something that is being offered freely. This is something to be overcome since it can perpetuate the idea that massage is an exclusive profession, done only by experts.

A genuine inhibition for friends and acquaintances arises from the conflict between intimacy and detachment. For good reasons, professionals tend not to treat their spouses, not that there need be any practical difficulty; what is unexpected is the paradoxical detachment and intimacy of massage.

111

Because a massage partner is not relaxing with you but through you, it can be alarming for your intimates to be aware of an unusual distance developing. For this reason, when partners are being chosen in the early sessions of a massage course, it is important that there must be freedom to reject a partnership offered, without an individual feeling this as a negative rejection – it can be that someone feels too strong an attraction rather than the opposite.

For a non-professional attempting to start a practice, bartering may be the best way. If someone has something that you feel is a good trade for your treatment, make an offer. On talking over a particular problem someone may be having in getting practice, we often find that rather than friends' reticence to be massaged (most are willing to a degree), the answer lies in the clarity of the massager's approach.

BELOW WHEN MASSAGING FRIENDS OR RELATIVES, SOME DETACHMENT IS REQUIRED ON THE PART OF THE PRACTITIONER.

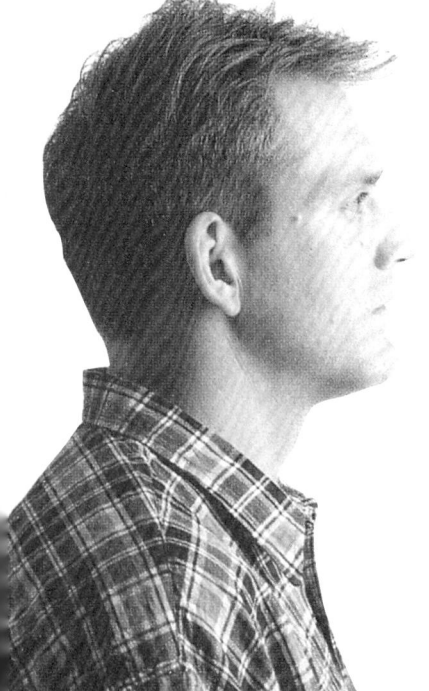
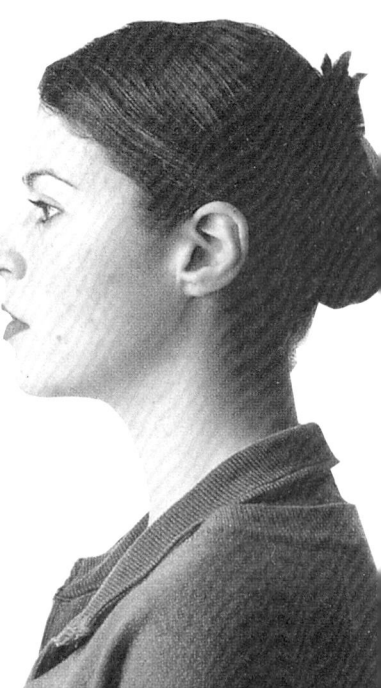

MASSAGE AND SEXUALITY

A major problem to be encountered sooner or later in practice, is how we reconcile our sexuality with the physicality of massage. This is not a unique problem since research has suggested that the subject of sex occupies much adult thinking time.

Sexual issues can arise in all human encounters, and quite naturally we have come to terms with them in reality of a treatment session. Just as in other life situations, the beginning of clearing away any sexual ambiguity in massage starts with the awareness of our own individual sexual consciousness. If this consciousness is a little dormant, you can be sure that it will awaken as your interest in massage grows. This can come as a shock to promising massagers, and misinterpretation may cause a retreat; even if you consider your attitude already enlightened, it is soon put to the test.

It is not always possible to know when a personal encounter is becoming sexualized. Many sexual responses take place at sub-conscious levels, and while your massage is intended to be a pleasurable experience, you may never know the quality of the sensation your partner is experiencing. From the point of view of this book, however, although the whole of a person's body may be regarded as sexual, the reproductive organs are not included in massage. In a class discussion group, many women massagers said they felt comfortable about sexuality being part of the massage experience. One man agreed, but when asked if this would include his male partners, he wasn't so sure. Some women in the group felt that the problem could be minimized by only working with partners of their own sex.

While it is very important to feel comfortable with your partner, in your early practice it may not be helpful to exclude people because of gender; massage offers an opportunity of honestly addressing sexuality, and your partner's embarrassment or naivete may only be mirroring your own. Sexual expression can also be representative – of anger, fear and other distress – and your honest attitude is just as important as your skill and attention in treatments.

Good massage engages the sensual aspect of our sexuality although this is not necessarily clear for first-time partners. People who are well controlled in daily life can be surprised at the depth of gentle massage; some may interpret new sensations as alarming, feeling the movement of their tensions as more chaotic than relaxing. From their position, a partner may find it hard not to feel that you are provoking these changes rather than facilitating them. It is the sensual element that forms the basis of unspoken rapport in massage, and for experienced practitioners it is regarded as an important aspect of the therapeutic relationship.

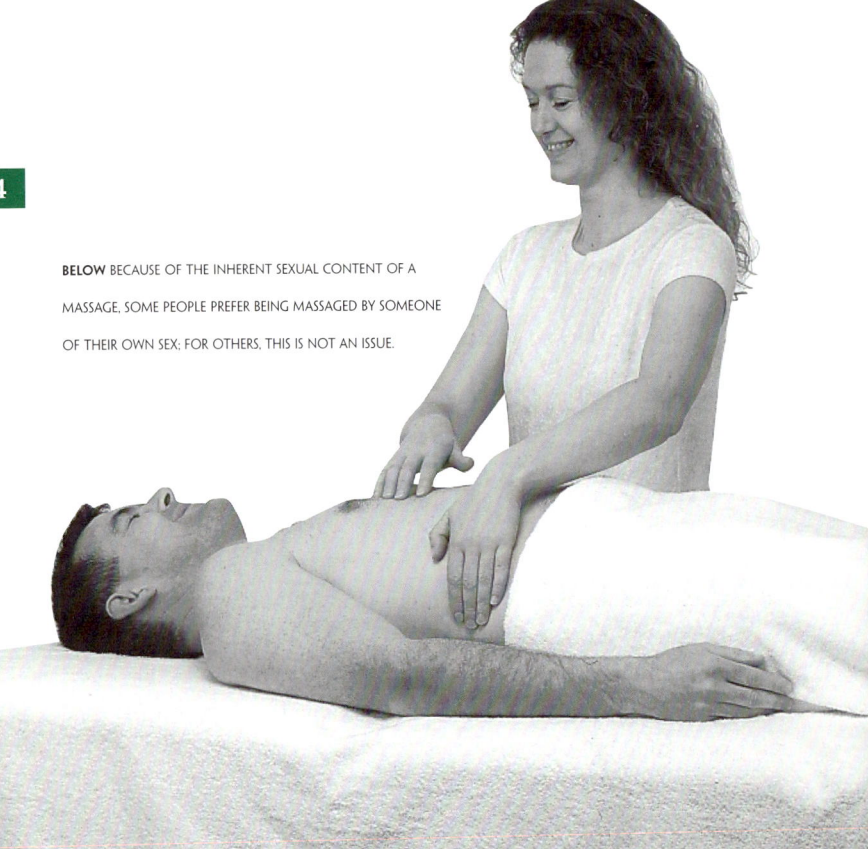

BELOW BECAUSE OF THE INHERENT SEXUAL CONTENT OF A MASSAGE, SOME PEOPLE PREFER BEING MASSAGED BY SOMEONE OF THEIR OWN SEX; FOR OTHERS, THIS IS NOT AN ISSUE.

TURNING PROFESSIONAL

If you have relieved someone's headache by massage, you are likely to attribute this to the methods you have used, which will have lessened the tension in the neck muscles. If you are using massage to help someone cope with a condition that has been acutely diagnosed, such as asthma or hypertension, you are more likely to be deploying massage's general effects of relaxation and reassurance.

The beneficial massages that have been described in this book, while undoubtedly therapeutic, are available to most beginners. Many people, with the briefest of training have shown a natural capacity to massage.

Physiotherapists need special training because their career directs them towards medical conditions and complications outside the scope of this book. In contrast, everyday massage aims to help prevent medical problems arising.

In your early practice, massage itself allows you to 'learn as you go', but at some point your successes will begin to activate your real curiosity about what's really going on – this is when you may feel like pursuing a professional course. There are many approaches to a formal study of massage although not all, surprisingly, emphasize the humanistic element.

FORMAL TRAINING

A professional course will involve examination, and the more 'natural' massagers find this an unappealing prospect. In order to achieve accreditation, however, it is generally accepted that a student should be able to impress favourably an examiner, who acts as a representative on behalf of future clients. At this stage the practitioner should be able to show style in handling rather than expertise, and be able to articulate the rationale for the treatment and the explanation of its effects.

Many serious massage students are those individuals who are looking for a change in their career or, more often, mature people who

115

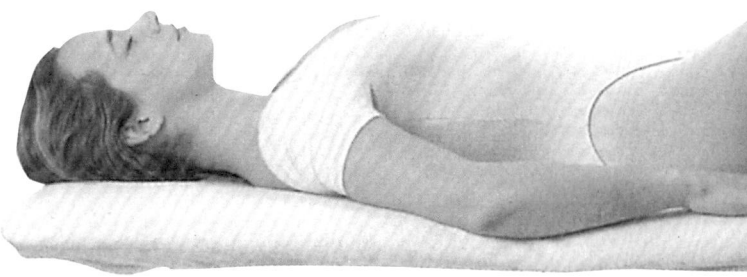

have sensed that in spite of having no clinical background, massage is just right for them. Increasingly, however, established professionals from the health field, such as nurses, home visitors and remedial teachers are finding that they can incorporate supportive massage into their work.

MASSAGE SCHOOLS

There are many independent schools of massage offering a wide variety of depth in method of study. Tutorials usually take place at weekends, allowing part-time attendance for practical coaching and guidance on study and learning methods.

Some courses are self-examined, where tutors assess the student on the technique or school of thought that they uphold; others are linked into wider professional organizations.

The Independent Examination Council (ITEC) combines both methods, offering a modulated examination system, where practitioners can move through basic massage therapy to aroma-therapy, injuries, nutrition, reflexology and sports exercise. This allows you to build up a practice gradually, offering general treatments from the beginning and adding to your expertise as you gain in experience.

The School of Complementary Therapies in Exeter offers an established post-graduate programme for massage therapists. This school also provides a professional association of graduates.

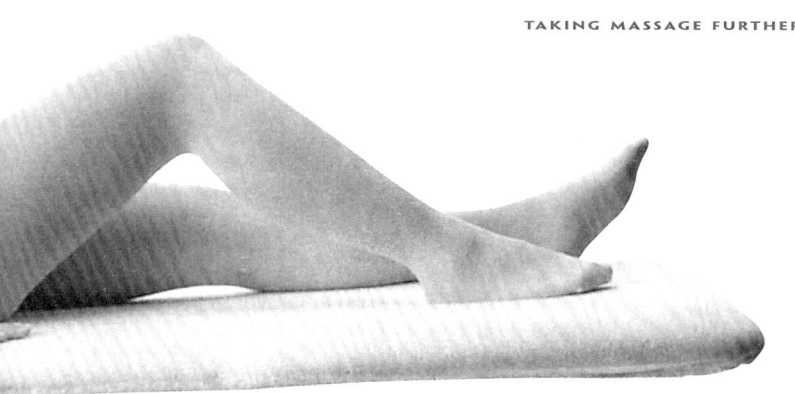

For readers wishing to practise massage outside the UK, I recommend the *International Massage & Bodywork Resource Guide*, published annually in the USA. This is a unique directory that lists schools, associations and laws relating to massage in 10 countries.

Some practitioners need guidance on the interactional aspects of massage, and if this has not been covered to your satisfaction in training, your local university may offer a counselling course, or might advise on a trainer.

It is important to realize that your training course is merely the preliminary to the practice of massage. The word "practice" is used within professions to make clear that a practitioner does not begin perfect but uses work experience to develop, discover and refine their initial burst of enthusiasm.

CHOOSING THE RIGHT COURSE

When choosing a course, be aware of what is being offered or promised; you should expect clear instruction, access to your tutor's professional experience and much encouragement to help organize your own plans, including post-graduate supervision.

Your massage school will be able to put you in contact with a professional organization for insurance purposes, but for most people, the end of their massage course brings with it the feeling they are now on their own. This has to be, of course, and a practice grows from the individual effort, frustrations and sudden inspirations of the individual.

If for any reason you are unable to keep contact with your school or have no fellow practitioners nearby, make friends with other professionals, share problems and difficult cases with anyone you feel you can trust, and avoid at all costs the isolation that can occur in both the quietest and busiest of practices.

There is an attitude, even among 'alternative' schools that only trained professionals are competent to treat others, but as I hope to have indicated throughout the book, massage is a human rather than technical experience. It belongs to our senses, like the talent to cook a satisfying meal that does not poison our guests or to be able to teach a friend to swim safely. If you decide, however, to formalize your interest in massage through a training course, I trust that your transition will be an integrated one – retaining the human touch while developing the responsibilities of professionalism.

In conclusion I offer every encouragement to you and your partners to follow the suggestions in this book and to be inspired to contribute to health and pleasure, and to continue to enjoy the giving and receiving of massage.

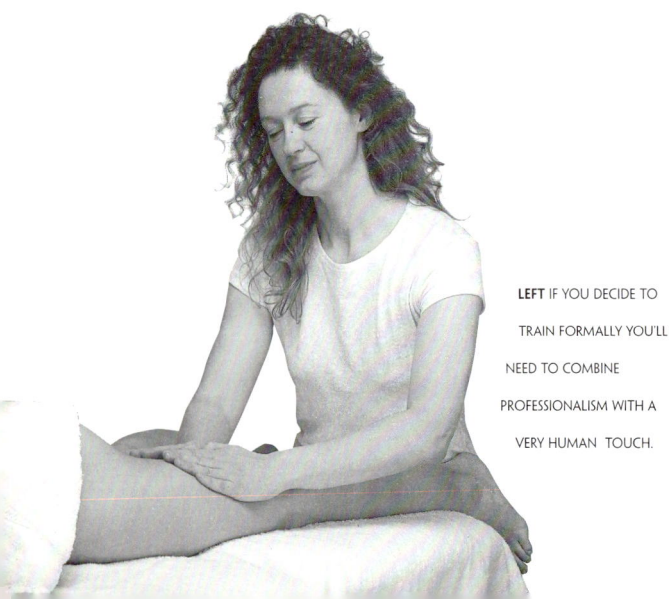

LEFT IF YOU DECIDE TO TRAIN FORMALLY YOU'LL NEED TO COMBINE PROFESSIONALISM WITH A VERY HUMAN TOUCH.

USEFUL ADDRESSES

For a list of schools offering the ITEC examination system write to:
The International Therapy Examination Council.

EUROPE

The International Therapy
Examination Council
10/11 Heathfield Terrace
Chiswick
London W4 4JE
Great Britain

Massage Therapy Institute of
Great Britain
PO Box 276
London NW2 4NR
Great Britain

For Post Graduate Training in
Massage contact:
The School of Complementary
Therapies
38 South Street
Exeter EX1 1ED
Great Britain

International Federation of
Aromatherapists
Stamford House
2–4 Chiswick High Road
London W4 1TH
Great Britain

AUSTRALASIA

Association of Massage
Therapists
3/33 Denham Street
Bondai
New South Wales NSW 2026
Australia

New Zealand Association of
Therapeutic Massage
Practitioners
PO Box 375
Hamilton
New Zealand

International Federation of
Aromatherapists
83 Riverdale Road
Hawthorn
Victoria 3122
Australia

NORTH AMERICA

American Massage Therapy
Association
820 Davis Street
Suite 100
Evanston
Illinois 60201-4444
USA
Tel: 1 708 864 0123
Fax: 1 708 864 1178

International Association of
Infant Massage
PO Box 438
Elma
New York 14059-0438
USA
Tel: 1 716 652 9789
Fax: 1 716 652 1990

International Massage
Association
3000 Connecticut Avenue NW
Apt 102
Washington, DC 20008
USA
Tel: 1 202 387 6555
Fax: 1 202 332 0531

National Association of Massage
Therapy
PO Box 1400
Westminster
Colorado 80030-1400
USA
Tel: 1 800 776 6268

American Aromatherapy
Association
PO Box 3679
South Pasadena
California 91031
USA
Tel: 818 457 1742

The Resource Guide can be
obtained from:
Noah Publishing
P0 Box 1500
Davis
CA 95617-1500
USA

GLOSSARY

Anatomy: the science of the shape and structure of the body and its parts. Initially daunting for serious massage students, they have the advantage of learning the living anatomy of partners as they learn to massage.

Artery: a tube-like vessel that carries blood away from the heart to the rest of the body.

Arthritis: inflammation of the structures within a skeletal joint.

Autonomic Nervous System: explains how the involuntary or unconscious functions, like breathing and digestion are controlled. The ANS has two complementary aspects: sympathetic nerves, concerned with stimulating, energetic action (speeding up); and parasympathetic nerves, which inhibit (slow down). Through these mechanisms the body's internal environment is kept in harmony.

Biceps: a muscle that has two points of attachment to a bone, e.g., the calf muscle, which can be felt behind the knee. Three points give Triceps: at the back of the upper arm: four points for Quadriceps, on the front of the thigh.

121

Central Nervous System: the actions of the nerves of the body that comprise the brain, spinal cord and peripheries. The CNS is characterized as controlling the conscious and deliberate movements of muscle and mind. Motor nerves relay instructions to the muscles to contract: sensor nerves record pain, heat, cold, etc. for the brain's interpretation. Nerves exit from spaces between the joints of the vertebral column and can be adversely affected by disorders of the joint.

Circulatory System: the movement of the blood around the body via the heart and its vessels, arteries and veins, and the lymphatics.

Couch: a custom-built table for massage treatment. It may be fixed or portable and should be designed to the appropriate height for the practitioner. (To test: stand sideways by the couch, arms by your side; flex your wrist so that your palm is now horizontal – this is the recommended couch height for you.)

Diagnosis: recognition of which disease a person has.

Diaphragm: the dome-like muscle that separates the contents of the chest from the abdomen. The diaphragm's active function is to assist full working of the lungs, while rhythmically massaging the digestive organs.

Dermis: the true skin, lying just beneath the outermost protective layer. The skin retains delicate sensitivity while forming an effective waterproof and thermal barrier for the body.

Endocrine System: describes the influence of hormones on the body. Hormones are chemical messengers, concentrated in glands strategically placed around the body. At critical times in our development, hormones are released directly into the bloodstream to bring about subtle changes in functioning.

Exudate: fluid blood containing an increased number of white blood cells that flows quickly to an injured area to begin the healing process.

122

Fibrositis: inflammation of the covering of the muscles, arising from excess tension or injury.

Hypertension: abnormal and undesirably high blood pressure.

Hypotension: low blood pressure. Not usually regarded as particularly unhealthy.

Immobilization: placing the body in such a position so as to minimize strain, especially if injured. Examples: resting a flexed knee over a pillow; placing the arm in a sling.

Insertion: the end of a muscle that is attached to the bone it intends to move. Example: the main calf muscle inserts on to the heel bone and by pulling on it, points the foot.

Inversion: to turn outside in.

Lymphatic System: a complementary circulation that parallels the venous return. Lymph, which is the water drained from tissues, together with disinfecting white blood cells, washes through from the peripheral body, cleansing and tidying en route back to the upper chest where it returns to the whole blood just before entry to the heart. The lymph is periodically drained as it passes through nodes, conveniently placed in crevices of the body: behind the knee, in the groin, under the arms, etc. The nodes also contain extra-powerful cleansing cells, lymphocytes, which can be transferred to the lymph in transit for emergencies of accident or illness.

Massage: manipulation of the soft tissues of the body for therapeutic purposes. Records of forms of massage have been recorded in all cultures from the earliest times.

Partner: someone who agrees to be massaged or exchange massage.

Posture: efficient alignment of the skeleton relative to any position but usually associated with upright stance. Posture can also mean attitude, which suggests that positioning has emotional and physical components.

Practitioner: one who gives massage professionally or with a committed interest.

Prone: facing downwards.

Psychology: the study of thought, emotion and behaviour, distinct from psychiatry, which is a medical speciality which treats diseases of the 'mind'.

Quadriceps: see Biceps.

Reflex: involuntary contraction of a muscle resulting from an unexpected stimulus. Occurs as in the 'tickling' mistake of a massage stroke that is too sudden or deep.

Rheumatism: formerly used for general forms of arthritis.

Sciatica: inflammation of the sciatic nerve, which runs from the lower back, behind the leg all the way underneath the foot. Sciatica often accompanies disorders of the vertebrae when these are misaligned or compressed.

Slipped Disc: a misnomer for a pressurized intervertebral disc (usually lumbar). The disc, which is made up of a cushion-like material, cannot actually slip but sometimes protrudes and interferes with the nerves exiting the spine. Discs are not 'put back in' even by the most exotic techniques, but are released by support and gentle traction.

Specialist: a practitioner with a concentrated approach, usually well experienced but in danger of 'finding out more and more about less and less'.

Stress: an excessive, unrelieved cycle of tension. Distinct from strain, which is self-regulating (something is hurting and we usually 'stop'), stress may be harder to recognize subjectively.

Tendon: the fibres at a muscle's end that attach it to a bone. Overuse of a muscle may inflame the tendon, producing tendonitis.

Therapy: literally 'to care for' and accompany a person in their illness. Parallel of patient, ('receptive to healing').

Traction: lengthening of the spine, usually from external stretch. Spontaneous traction occurs throughout the spine on each exhalation.

Trauma: literally 'wound', having physical and psychological consequences.

Treatment: what the therapist offers: a 'treat'.

Triceps: *See* Biceps.

Vasoconstriction: diminution of the smaller arteries; pallor; the effect of cold water on the skin's blood vessels.

Vasodilatation: expansion of the smaller arteries; blushing; the effect of alcohol on the skin's blood vessels (we feel 'warm'). The rapidly alternating vasoconstriction and vasodilation of the abdomen's tiny blood vessels when we are nervous gives the sensation of 'butterflies'.

Vein: a tube-like vessel that conducts blood back to the heart. Relatively superficial, the veins can be seen and felt, especially when varicose, full of pressure and struggling to overcome the effects of gravity.

Recommended Reading

Amadon, A. *The Fold Out Atlas of the Human Body*, Bonanza Books, 1984.

Asimov, I. *The Human Body*, New American Library, 1963.

Bertherat, T. *The Body Has Its Reasons*, Heinemann, 1988.

Bettany, C. *The Thinking Body*, Anow Books, 1989.

Curtis Shears, C. *Nutrition Science & Health Education*, Nutrition Science Institute, 1978.

Freud, S. *The Psychopathology of Everyday Life*, Penguin, 1975.

Hauser, G.B. *Better Eyes Without Glasses*, Faber, 1956.

Ingham, E. *Reflexology Stories the Feet Can Tell*, Ingam Publishing Inc., 1984.

Knott, B.S. & Voss, E. *Proprioceptive Neuromuscular Technique*, Hoeber-Harper, 1962.

Lederman, E. *Good Health Through Natural Therapy*, Kogan Page, 1976.

Liechti, E. *Health Essentials: Shiatsu*, Element, 1992.

Lewis, S. *An Anatomical Wordbook*, Butterworth-Heinemann, 1990.

Li-Hui, J. & Zhao – Xiang, J. *Pointing Therapy*, Shandong Science Press, 1984.

Masters, P. *Osteopathy for Everyone*, Penguin, 1988.

Siegel, A. *Polarity Therapy*, Prism Press, 1987.

Thomson, C. L. *Hydrotherapy – Water and Nature Cure*, Kingston Publications, 1970.

Wildwood, C. *New Perspectives: Aromatherapy*, Element, 1999.

Wirhed, R. *Athletic Ability and the Anatomy of Motion*, Wolfe, 1984.

INDEX